1/c

Health Care Education

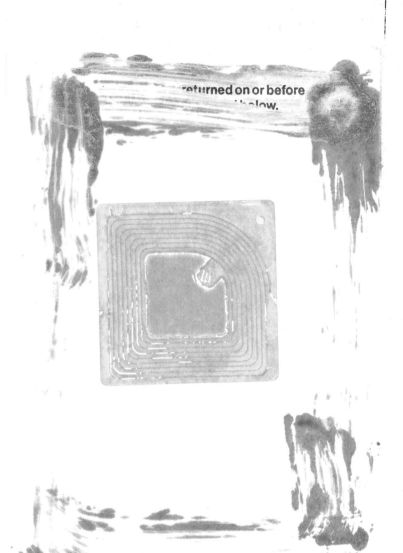

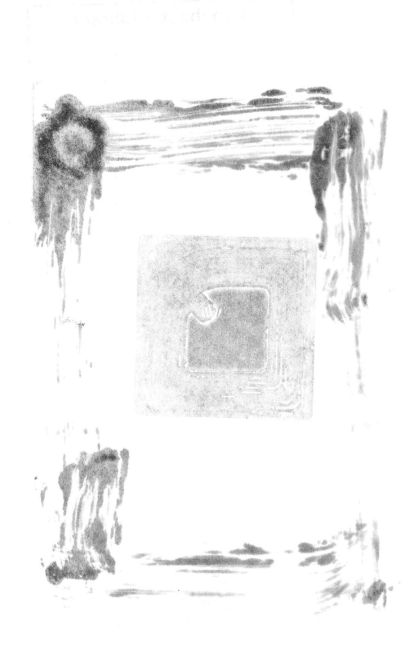

Health Care Education

THE CHALLENGE OF THE MARKET

Edited by

John Humphreys

and

Francis M. Quinn

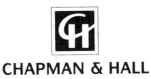

CHAPMAN & HALL

London · Glasgow · Weinheim · New York · Tokyo · Melbourne · Madras

Published by Chapman & Hall, 2–6 Boundary Row London SE1 8HN, UK

Chapman & Hall, 2–6 Boundary Row, London SE1 8HN, UK

Blackie Academic & Professional, Wester Cleddens Road, Bishopbriggs, Glasgow G64 2NZ, UK

Chapman & Hall GmbH, Pappelallee 3, 69469 Weinheim, Germany

Chapman & Hall USA, One Penn Plaza, 41st Floor, New York NY 10119, USA

Chapman & Hall Japan, ITP-Japan, Kyowa Building, 3F, 2-2-1 Hirakawacho, Chiyoda-ku, Tokyo 102, Japan

Chapman & Hall Australia, Thomas Nelson Australia, 102 Dodds Street, South Melbourne, Victoria 3205, Australia

Chapman & Hall India, R. Seshadri, 32 Second Main Road, CIT East, Madras 600 035, India

First edition 1994

© 1994 Chapman & Hall

Typeset in Times 10/12 pt by EXPO Holdings, Malaysia
Printed in Great Britain by T.J. Press (Padstow) Ltd, Padstow, Cornwall

ISBN 0 412 57500 0

A catalogue record for this book is available from the British Library

∞ Printed on Permanent acid-free text paper, manufactured in accordance with ANSI/NISO Z39.48–1992 and ANSI/NISO Z39.48–1984 (Permanence of Paper).

Contents

Contributors

Bill Bailey
Associate Head, School of Post Compulsory Education and Training, University of Greenwich, London, UK

Dai Hall
Professional Liaison and Development Director, School of Post Compulsory Education and Training, University of Greenwich, London, UK

John Humphreys
Head, School of Post Compulsory Education and Training, University of Greenwich, London, UK

Ray Land
Senior Lecturer, Educational Development Unit, Napier University, Edinburgh, UK

Francis M. Quinn
Director of Health Care Education, University of Greenwich, London, UK

Bobbi Ramsammy
Dean, Faculty of Health, University of Greenwich, London, UK

Stephanie Stanwick
Principal Commissioner (Priority and Community Care), West Kent Health Authority, Kent, UK

Val Thomson
Head of Division, Advanced Studies and Midwifery, Sussex and Kent Institute, Brighton, UK

Alan Walker
Director of Education, Chartered Society of Physiotherapy, London, UK

Preface

Sometime in the 1980s, Norbert Singer, the then Director of Thames Polytechnic, became interested in the idea of becoming involved in nurse education. Project 2000 had been published. In those days, there were three qualified nurses in the Polytechnic: all in the School of Post Compulsory Education and Training, and all involved in the training of nurse tutors. Knowing this, he telephoned the Head of School: 'Take an interest in this', he said, 'Let's see how far it can go'. Singer had perceived the possibility of a new market – a major opportunity for his institution. Whereas we had been active in various minor collaborations before, after that telephone call the development of health care education became a strategic priority.

Now Thames Polytechnic is the University of Greenwich. We have a Faculty of Health with P2000 and 100+ staff; a major interest in physiotherapy training through a national agreement with the Chartered Society of Physiotherapy; the UK's first operational ENB Higher Award with Princess Alexandra and Newham College of Nursing and Midwifery and 1000+ students working for Greenwich awards through *Nursing Times* Open Learning. These developments are indicative of the scale and scope of recent changes in health care education.

Through this period of frenetic and exciting development we, like many others around the country, have been reflecting on the pace, nature and significance of these national changes. Our school's background has been in vocational and professional education generally and we have probably benefited in our deliberations from the fact that one of us is an 'insider' in relation to health care education (Francis M. Quinn) while the other is not (John Humphreys).

In applying our school's generic knowledge of professional education to the health care area, we have inevitably been drawn to comparisons between health care education and the other post compulsory sectors of education and training. In making these comparisons, we have come to believe that something interesting and unprecedented is happening in health care education.

Essentially a national experiment in professional education is under way. In this (largely unplanned) experiment, a new NHS organization provides a market for education. In this market, corporate colleges (Universities) increasingly provide services for 'corporate' employers (NHS trusts). Although health regions currently devise the rules for this market, there is no national funding mechanism, only the broad guidelines of 'Working Paper 10'. As a subset of a wider debate, we will describe how the education market positions the old 'immovable object' of the health care professions against the new 'unstoppable force' of the new NHS trusts. We do not know where these changes will finally lead but we already perceive radical change. Collectively the chapters of this volume represent an analysis of the implications and effects of the new market for education.

We hope that the combination of analyses and case studies will make the book useful and interesting to actual and prospective teachers, managers and practitioners involved in health care education on either side of the market. In particular those interested in nursing, midwifery, professions supplementary to medicine, and complementary medicine may find issues discussed that are of direct relevance to the challenges they are currently facing.

At another level, however, the analytical and case study chapters can be seen in the context of a central thesis that provides an organizing principle for the book. We believe that the new circumstances of health care education have already triggered radical change in the practice of education. We have described this change loosely as a paradigm shift in which an old orthodoxy is being deserted by practitioners of education inclined to survive the new environment.

Broadly speaking, the book is divided into two halves. The first five chapters constitute a consideration of the orthodox paradigm of health care education (Chapters 1 and 2) followed by a series of case studies (Chapters 3, 4 and 5) which in varying degrees are seen to be incompatible with it. The second half is concerned with the causes and effects of change, and includes an analysis of the market for health care education (Chapter 6), the position of colleges in relation to client and other organizations (Chapter 7), aspects of the internal structure of colleges (Chapter 8) and finally an attempt to review the main thesis of the book and to articulate aspects of the newly-emerging paradigm in more detail (Chapter 9). Each chapter includes an editors' introduction which positions the chapter in the context of our thesis. Table 0.1 shows the structure of the book in relation to its main thesis.

The idea for the book arose not just through our curriculum and management development work. The extent to which the ideas and issues are being faced on a national scale has been revealed to us at conferences and through our consultancy activities in curriculum development, management and marketing for a number of colleges. Furthermore our consultancy work has included regional level projects on the development of market systems for linking quality to contracting. We have therefore been active on both sides of the education market and we must thank our client organizations for giving us these opportunities.

Most of all however, we must recognize and acknowledge all those staff within the School of Post Compulsory Education and Training, whose original work on credit systems (cited in various chapters) provided the foundation for our various subsequent developments in health care education.

Table 0.1 Diagrammatic representation of the structure of the book in relation to its main thesis

Chapter	1	Establishes the main thesis of paradigm change in Health Care Education
Chapter	2	Considers the orthodox paradigm and its problems
Chapter	3	Provides evidence of change
	4	through case studies which
	5	demonstrate inconsistencies with the established paradigm
Chapter	6	Provides analysis of the causes
	7	of change and effects
	8	on college structure and management
Chapter	9	Articulates elements of a new paradigm including a new model for curriculum development implicit in current innovative education practice

For help with the production and editing of the manuscript, we must thank Jan Borders of the University of Greenwich.

It would be conventional at this point to thank our wives, but in fact they have successful careers of their own and are much too busy to spend time helping their husbands figure out the esoteric complexities of health care education. However, making them cups of tea has sometimes helped clarify our minds.

Health care education: towards a corporate paradigm

1

John Humphreys and Francis M. Quinn

Editors' introduction

In this chapter the concept of paradigm destabilization is applied as a metaphor for the educational revolution consequent upon the introduction of market forces into health care education. The status of UKCC Project 2000 as a radical educational reform is discussed, and the basic thesis of the book is defined.

INTRODUCTION

In 1962, Thomas Kuhn published his seminal work on the structure of scientific revolutions. In it, he argued that philosophers of science had been misled in their analysis of the nature of the endeavour. In contrast to the then conventional view of science as objective reality assembled through disinterested experiment, Kuhn, through historical analysis, saw only communities of scientists acting like human beings. They were often reluctant to change their ways, precious about their theories and inclined to dogma. Most of their time was spent trying to solve puzzles set in a dominant conceptual framework of received beliefs which the community acknowledged as supplying the foundation for its practice. These received beliefs he called the 'paradigm'. It enshrined values, methods of work and fundamental concepts which provided the basis of explanation. The dogma of the paradigm, he claimed, is maintained through social pressure and education. If someone discovers or does something inconsistent with the paradigm, it is normally considered the problem of the individual, not the paradigm. Perhaps the experiment was flawed or the technique inaccurate or maybe the scientist wasn't quite up to it. Inevitably the quality of the work is questioned. In any event, no scientific group could practise its trade without its received beliefs and, in this context, education and training must initiate the new recruit into the paradigm. Textbooks serve their purpose by focusing on achievements which support the paradigm. What point is there in disseminating those data which, since unexplainable, must clearly be problematic?

From time to time, however, something may destabilize the paradigm. Perhaps an unavoidable accumulation of evidence apparently refuting central tenets. Perhaps a moment of new insight amounting to genius. Such events must be enormously persuasive since the defence of the paradigm is strong. After all, careers are at stake; strongly held values are questioned and dogma is more re-assuring than confusion. Such events imply radical change and Kuhn therefore identified the replacement of one paradigm with the next as 'revolution'.

Since its publication, Kuhn's work has been widely discussed, widely applied and widely misused. In this chapter, we will probably misuse it a bit more. However, we will not do this naively. Kuhn's ideas concern science, an endeav-our which is different from and conducted in a less complex environment than health care or health care education. We do not therefore claim any direct corre-spondence between the two, but we do recognize some analogous situations, and from them some insights that we wish to bring to bear on the current state of health care education.

In the first place, Kuhn's work carried a technical definition of revolution which we find useful. Revolution in the sense that we use the term need not be fast (although often it will be) and may not generate much interest outside the professional community (although it may receive press coverage). But it must be radical and therefore, to a large degree, incompatible with what went before. In this way, we can distinguish between reform – in which what went before is re-moulded (or reformed) – and revolution in which new methods, concepts and even values (collectively a new paradigm) replace earlier ones with which they may have little relationship. Our revolution then is simply a fundamental change which has, and is, radically shifting the practice of health care education.

Although wide-ranging in its coverage, the central thesis of this book is that a set of established values, received beliefs and methods of operating are in the process of being overturned. Since we regard these values, beliefs and methods as, to a degree, dogma, we are drawn to a Kuhnian analogy. Essentially in health care education, a long-standing curriculum paradigm is being deserted by educa-tional practitioners.

Kuhn showed that what might be called professional communities can operate in ways less idealistic than they sometimes claim. Commonly scientists, while believing fervently in objective truth, in fact sacrifice this high ideal to a dog-matic commitment to favoured ideas. If scientists can do this type of thing, then so can health care professionals and so can educationalists. In those interim (rev-olutionary) periods between paradigms, Kuhn described practitioners arguing vehemently for one or the other side. In fact, in these communities such changes can provoke severe criticism by practitioners of the work of contemporaries. In education we perceive current debates relating orthodoxy to 'standards' as one of many manifestations of this interim period.

Kuhn's concept of paradigm was somewhat problematic from the start. Masterman (1970) found that, in introducing the idea, Kuhn had used 'paradigm' in at least 21 different senses. Since 1962, the idea of paradigm has received abundant analysis which it is not our intention to review here. Suffice it to say that Kuhn's paradigms have been extrapolated beyond their scientific origins across a range of intellectual endeavours. Although still problematic in various respects, there is no question that Kuhn's ideas on paradigms and revolution have proved useful in analyses of the development of ideas and the behaviour of communities of practitioners beyond those working in the sciences.

However it is by no means clear that the original Kuhnian concepts of paradigm and revolution always apply. The general Kuhnian progression may not, for example, apply where there is no universally accepted paradigm to overthrow (Bottomore, 1971, argued this of sociology). Sociologists can also argue that there was little originality in Kuhn's views of education. Education as a process of socialization is not a new idea; Simpson (1967), for example, showed how pre-registration nursing courses effectively socialized new recruits into the profession (Chapter 9).

Before committing ourselves to paradigms for the purposes of our book, we must ask the question as to whether health care educators as a professional community do in fact hold a paradigm that fairly universally informs their practice. Schein and Kommers (1972) made a distinction between the practice of professions and the theoretical paradigms which underpin practice. In doing this they distinguished between professions, which they considered to achieve a high degree of consensus on underlying paradigms (engineering and law) from others in which consensus was not apparent (teaching and clinical psychology).

We consider such analyses to be anachronistic in that they imply a fairly static interface between theory and practice in professions, which the work of Schon (1991) and others have shown in fact to be a dynamic and fuzzy distinction involving a considerable degree of interaction. For our current purposes we would like to postulate that professions can operate on the basis of paradigms of practice rather than simply practice on the basis of underlying theoretical paradigms. Such paradigms of practice may be compatible with a range of theories, models, etc., but carry certain fundamental value and method commitments. This point is considered further in Chapter 2.

A perennial problem with paradigms is that, whereas many consider them a useful idea, once an attempt is made to describe one in any definitive way the difficulties originally identified by Masterman reappear. A recent example of dispute over what is or is not a paradigm can be seen in the area of social psychology. In this case Harre (1993) has defended his position that a paradigm shift has indeed occurred in social psychology (challenged by Farr, 1993) by referring to Fleck's original expression of 'thought style' from which Kuhn derived his idea of the paradigm. Fleck used this phrase to indicate an idea of commonality in a more loosely structured field than paradigms have come to represent.

Since there is a danger that such disputes would be a hindrance (and peripheral) to the main purpose of this book, we will sidestep the issue by arguing analogy with, rather than correspondence to, strictly Kuhnian paradigms. Essentially we have found Kuhn's insight illuminating in our analysis and although our paradigms may be better described as 'thought styles' in fact the more we consider the manifestation of change the more we are drawn back to Kuhn.

As Mulkay (1991) observed, Kuhn's paradigms imply an endeavour characterized not by intellectual openness but by the intellectual closure of practitioners who, while they may generate and discuss many theories and models, rarely bring into question basic assumptions. Chapter 2 reviews some of the

Table 1.1 Some features of two conflicting paradigms of health care education

	Destabilized orthodox paradigm	*Incipient new paradigm*
Primary concerns	1. The profession 2. The patient	1. The corporate organization 2. The student
Ideologies	Various	Instrumental
Values	Patient as client of education	Employer as client of education
	Student as moral responsibility	Student as consumer
	Education as entry to profession	Education for strategic development
	Student as putative professional	Student as workforce supply
	Education as in-house	Purchaser/provider split
	Quality as intellectual rigour	Quality as fitness for purpose
	Curriculum as established practice	Curriculum as product
Methods of Work – Curriculum derivation	Professional regulation Epistemological analysis Education-led curriculum development	Market demands Training needs analysis Market-led curriculum development
– Process	Teacher as socialization agent	Teacher as change agent
Fundamental concepts	Courses Coherence (as internal to course) Progression (as enshrined in specified sequence)	Flexible learning programmes Coherence (as internal to students) Progression (as internal to students)

theories and models of curriculum commonly used by health care education and identifies an underlying assumption implied by their consistent neglect of employers. Yet for many practitioners of health care education, employers are now seen at the very centre of their activities (see, for example, Chapter 8). From our consideration of these two stances (reviewed in Chapter 9) we have identified two distinct 'thought styles' or paradigms, one orthodox and one new.

Table 1.1 summarizes our view of some aspects of the old and new paradigms. We position it here as an 'advance organizer' (Ausubel 1978) for the book but we will leave our detailed arguments until later (especially Chapters 2 and 9). Since we argue a current intermediate stage, neither paradigm is considered to correspond exactly to the existing situation. In the current confusion, elements of both paradigms are manifest (we hope the case studies illustrate this point).

CAUSES OF CHANGE

Textbooks can give us clues (we would not say evidence) as to the possible causes of the radical changes. In this respect omissions may be most important. We have so far failed to find a textbook of health care education that gives any serious consideration to the new employers of health care professionals. Even recent publications in educational journals or from statutory bodies consistently neglect NHS trusts; and from some publications it would be difficult to believe that they exist. Yet it is inconceivable that authors or statutory bodies are unaware of the significance for education of NHS trusts. In our view, this apparent inability to make the connection between employers and professional education reveals an inability of the existing paradigm to accommodate corporate-style employers. While such organizations increase their power and influence, the curriculum paradigm precludes anything but a superficial response. As the mismatch increases, so practitioners of education are deserting the established paradigm and so innovative case studies become inexplicable in conventional terms.

Over the last few years, a major preoccupation of health care educators has been the introduction of 'Project 2000' (UKCC, 1986) courses for the initial training of nurses. These courses differed from previous ones in that students became pre-service rather than in-service (i.e. when in clinical placement they were supernumerary to the necessary workforce). Additionally P2000 courses lead to higher education qualifications whereas most earlier pre-registration training had not.

The extent to which this development has dominated the minds of nurse educators is reflected by the avalanche of analyses and reports which are now available in the literature. However, in the context of professional education generally, P2000 does not constitute a radical reform. In identifying nurse education as higher education, and students as supernumerary, P2000 simply brought nurse education into line with the education of many other professional groups. Although representing a real challenge to health care education providers, there are few new educational principles implied or enshrined within it. Although often represented as a highly significant educational reform, the real significance of P2000 is not to education but to the profession. It constitutes more than anything a reform of the profession of nurse. Through orthodox but changed education, P2000 has identified the nurse as different from before. It has profound implications for her/his position as a practitioner and in relation to other workers in the clinical environment. By virtue of its explicit link with HE awards, P2000 has recognized and consolidated the nurse's position as a 'professional' practitioner. It is, in short, an education-led reform of the profession of nurse and, although it radically changes the profession and raises many clinical and employment issues, solutions to the educational challenges of P2000 can be abstracted from many precedents, parallels and precursors in the domain of professional education. Seen in isolation P2000 may be radical for the profession, but in education terms it is not in itself revolutionary.

The true educational significance of P2000 is revealed when it is considered in the context of NHS reorganization. In order to create the internal market for health services, district health authorities (DHAs) have undergone a change of role. Whereas previously health services were provided by 'units' within DHAs, these units are now becoming independent NHS trusts. This enables Districts to take a role in the purchasing of health services (on behalf of patients) from NHS trusts. This purchaser–provider split constitutes the main element of the market. Since all transactions fall within the scope of the Department of Health, the market is considered to be 'internal'.

These general NHS reorganizations posed various issues for education. In the event, regional health authorities were given the initial responsibility for funding education through a process originally published by the Department of Health as Working Paper 10 (WP10). At this point the position of DHAs in relation to education became ambiguous. With colleges located within DHAs, districts were essentially providing regionally funded education services for those trusts from which they were purchasing health services. The anomalous nature of this position had, because of P2000, a ready-made solution. P2000 had driven colleges into close links with higher education. With strong links already developed, it therefore became inevitable that many colleges would incorporate into universities. After some prevarication, the NHS ruled out most other options and, at the time of writing, the process of incorporation of colleges into universities is widespread.

Thus, in the spirit of health service reorganization, an incipient market for education positions regional health authorities as purchasers of education services from higher education institutions. Unlike the internal market for health care provision, the education market has been created through the combined effects of relatively unrelated policy decisions, driven by much larger financial and other imperatives of NHS reform. Furthermore the education market lies across government departments and is therefore, for the moment at least, not entirely 'internal'.

Educational change, therefore, has been a consequence of larger reorganizations rather than any single coherent policy. In creating links between health care education and universities, P2000 provided a ready-made solution to an education problem posed by NHS reform, and this synergistic interaction between P2000 and NHS reorganization resulted in an education contracting system for which (as Chapter 7 argues) there are no precedents.

Paradoxically, then, we have the situation where P2000, much discussed as an educational reform, in fact carries limited educational novelty, while general NHS reform carries revolutionary implications for education. This book is about a revolution in the practice of health care education driven in the last analysis by the reorganization of the NHS.

For our present purposes a revolution can be considered to involve three distinct although chronologically overlapping elements – first, the established or orthodox paradigm; second, an interim period of relative confusion; and third, a new paradigm. We believe that there is now evidence of a significant departure from orthodoxy. Chapter 2 includes an analysis of this orthodoxy and asserts its demise. Chapters 3, 4 and 5 describe case studies, each of which illustrates a significant departure from earlier practice.

We also believe that health care education currently occupies an interim position in which the practice of education is more variable and volatile than before. This position seems an almost inevitable consequence of complex interactions between the different issues that health care education is currently addressing. On the one hand the move into higher education is in some institutions raising the prospect of academization, led by those universities more committed to theory than to professional practice. Meanwhile increasingly confident NHS trusts look for an educational contribution of skilled and reskilled practitioners to progress their strategic development. Somewhere between these two corporate sectors, statutory and professional bodies can be found trying to reconcile their twin desires of graduate status and professional focus – and of course these things are not incompatible.

We do not claim to know exactly which way things will go over the next few years. A critical factor will be the long-term location of the control of education funding and in particular the ways in which the market for education is managed. However, already some things have gone beyond the point where they can easily be reversed. On one side of the education market there are now NHS trusts and on the other (increasingly) universities. These two influential, independent and corporate sectors therefore represent the beginnings of a new stability in our otherwise changing educational environment. In these circumstances education would appear almost inevitably to be moving towards what we will call a corporate paradigm. This movement is the subject of our book.

Policy changes in education and training may create various dilemmas for education practitioners. While on one level they may need to review aspects of their current practice to anticipate or better accommodate the new environment, on another, conflicts may arise with regard to the moral and/or political issues that such changes may raise. The purpose of this book is not to address the latter issues. In particular it does not attempt a critique of the new situation and indeed we have avoided adopting any particular moral or political stance. Although we certainly hope to provoke a debate, we believe that a full critique should follow research into the actual effects of the new environment on education and its effectiveness.

Although in due course we intend to address the moral and political issues raised by these developments, our present purpose is simply to describe, analyse and inform, and in so doing to help practitioners of education address the practical dilemmas and challenges that the new environment creates.

REFERENCES

Ausubel, D. (1978) *Educational Psychology: A Cognitive View*, Holt, Rinehart & Winston, New York.

Bottomore, T.B. (1971) *Sociology: A Guide to Problems and Literature*, Unwin, London.

Farr, R. (1993) A devise is not a paradigm. *Psychologist*, **June**, 261–252.

Harre, R. (1993) Paradigms, experiment and the discursive turn. *Psychologist*, **June**, 263.

Kuhn, T. (1962) *The Structure of Scientific Revolutions*, University of Chicago Press, Chicago.

Masterman, M. (1970) The nature of a paradigm, in *Criticism and the Growth of Knowledge*, (ed. M. Lakatos and A. Musgrave), Cambridge University Press, Cambridge.

Mulkay, M. (1991) *Sociology of Science: A Sociological Pilgrimage* Open University Press, Milton Keynes.

Schein, E.H. and Kommers, D.W. (1972) *Professional Education : Some New Directions*, McGraw-Hill, London.

Schon, D.A. (1991) *The Reflective Practitioner How Professionals Think in Action*, Avebury, Aldershot.

Simpson, I.H. (1967) Patterns of socialization into professions: the case of student nurses. *Sociological Inquiry*, **37**, 47–54.

UKCC (United Kingdom Central Council for Nursing, Midwifery and Health Visiting) (1986) *Project 2000: A New Preparation for Practice*, UKCC, London.

Department of Health (1989) *Working for Patients, Education and Training*, Working Paper 10. HMSO, London.

The demise of curriculum

2

Francis M. Quinn

Editors' introduction

This chapter reviews the established canon of the orthodox curriculum paradigm which is described as largely school-derived and based on ideas of coherence and progression which are no longer universally applied.

Increasing departure from these established ideas has been caused by a process of 'professionalization' which has pushed health care education into the sphere of higher education and has resulted in exposure to credit schemes, APEL, etc., combined with the effects of WP10 funding.

Since the conventional approach has been characterized by inadequate relations between educators and service providers, the author asserts that a new paradigm must emerge in which education gives as much priority to employers as to students.

INTRODUCTION

Curriculum is the single most important concept in education, encompassing as it does all the activities normally included under the umbrella terms 'education' and 'training'. In health care education, as in other branches of education, teachers use established theories and models as the basis for curriculum development within their respective fields of study. However, the established models were developed for the education of children, and this orientation remains intact when curriculum models are adapted for use with adults in health care education, resulting in the omission of the employer/client entirely from the curriculum design process.

Furthermore, these orthodox curriculum theories and models tend to form a closed system, within which adaptations of the original models are developed but which leave the essential nature of the models unchanged. In this way, curriculum models and theories for adult education in general, and for health care education in particular have a face validity which on closer examination is found to be largely spurious. Using the term 'paradigm' in the sense in which it was defined in Chapter 1, it is my contention that these curriculum theories and models constitute an educational paradigm to which health care education is inextricably bound. This paradigm is so well entrenched that even the sea-changes occurring within the health service have had, as yet, only a minor impact upon it.

The aim of this chapter is to describe, analyse and destabilize the orthodox paradigm of health care education.

CURRICULUM: THE ESTABLISHED CANON

Definitions of curriculum

The first book on the subject, Franklin Bobbitt's *The Curriculum*, appeared in 1918 and curriculum theory has subsequently emerged as an established field of study within education. An examination of the literature, however, reveals that the concept of curriculum is by no means straightforward. There is wide variation between definitions and a number of writers (e.g. Lewis and Miel, 1972; Tanner and Tanner, 1980; Saylor, Alexander and Lewis, 1981) have attempted to categorize these. Four main interpretations of the concept emerge and these are given below, along with a range of definitions from the literature.

1. **Curriculum as objectives:** 'Any statement of the objectives of the school should be a statement of changes to take place in students' (Tyler, 1949).
2. **Curriculum as subject matter:** 'A curriculum is the offering of socially-valued knowledge, skills and attitudes made available to students through a variety of arrangements during the time they are at school, college or university' (Bell, 1973).
3. **Curriculum as student experiences:** 'Curriculum is all the learning which is planned and guided by the school whether it is carried on in groups or individually, inside or outside the school' (Kerr, 1968).
4. **Curriculum as opportunities for students:** 'A curriculum is all the educational opportunities encountered by students as a direct result of their involvement with an educational institution' (Quinn, 1988).

Skilbeck's (1984) categorization has considerable overlap with the previous one, but the aspect of culture is introduced:

1. Curriculum as a structure of forms and fields of knowledge;
2. Curriculum as a chart or map of the culture;
3. Curriculum as a pattern of learning activities;
4. Curriculum as a learning technology.

This categorization has been adapted by Beattie in his fourfold model of curriculum, described later in this chapter.

Other writers (e.g. Stenhouse, 1975; Saylor *et al.*, 1981) take a more generic view of the concept, seeing it as an overall plan or design for learning: 'Curriculum is an attempt to communicate the essential principles and features of an educational proposal in such a form that it is open to critical scrutiny and capable of effective translation into practice' (Stenhouse, 1975); 'Curriculum is a plan for providing sets of learning opportunities for persons to be educated' (Saylor *et al.*, 1981); 'Curriculum refers to the learning experiences of students, in so far as they are expressed or anticipated in educational goals and objectives, plans and designs for learning and the implementation of these plans and designs in school environments' (Skilbeck, 1984).

My own approach is very much in this vein. I like to think of the curriculum as a plan or design for education/training that addresses the following questions.

1. **Who is to be taught/will learn?** This is the consumer of the curriculum, i.e. the student, course member, colleague, etc. who will experience the curriculum.
2. **What is to be taught/learned?** This is about both the intentions and the content of the curriculum. Intentions may or may not be stated overtly, according to the education ideology underpinning the curriculum. Where outcomes, goals or objectives are overtly expressed, these statements also indicate to some extent the nature of the curriculum content. If the intentions are covert, then content is usually indicated by a list of topics in a syllabus.
3. **Why is it to be taught/learned?** This is the ideology of the curriculum, i.e. the beliefs and values that underpin the curriculum approach.
4. **How is it to be taught/learned?** This is the process of education, i.e. the teaching, learning and assessment approaches/opportunities available to the consumer.
5. **Where is it to be taught/learned?** This is the context of the curriculum, i.e. the faculty, department, school, college, campus, rooms, etc. It also refers to the place of a given curriculum within the range of awards of the education provider institution.
6. **When is it to be taught/learned?** This is the programming/timetabling of the curriculum, i.e. the length, pattern of attendance, etc.

The concept of curriculum has been further subdivided by some commentators and the more common subdivisions are 'official curriculum' – the curriculum laid down in the policy of the institution; 'actual curriculum' – the curriculum as implemented by teachers; 'hidden curriculum' – the attitudes and values transmitted by the teachers.

The field of curriculum studies comprises a number of concepts that tend to be used interchangeably within the literature, such as ideologies, theory and models. Some clarification of these terms is now required.

Curriculum ideologies

An individual's concept of the curriculum is shaped by the system of beliefs and values that s/he holds about education; in other words, the educational ideology to which s/he subscribes. A number of such educational ideologies have been identified (e.g. Davies, 1969; Scrimshaw, 1983), each with its own adherents who share common values and beliefs about the educational enterprise and whose views may conflict with those of adherents to other ideologies. The essential features of the prevailing curriculum ideologies are outlined below.

Conservative/classical humanism

These ideologies focus on the nation, and view education as the transmission of the cultural heritage of a nation; key values are stability and a sense of continuity with the past. Curricula are differentiated for the elite and the non-elite and the curriculum is subject-centred and teacher-dominated. Motivation is extrinsic, with an emphasis on discipline.

Democratic/liberal humanism

The emphasis here is on the role of education in the creation of a common democratic culture, with educational opportunity for all. Key values are quality, relevance and lifelong education. Curricula are common-core and teacher–pupil negotiation features as a teaching strategy.

Romantic/progressivism

These ideologies see education as meeting the needs, aspirations and personal growth of the individual. They emphasize the process of learning by experience, group discovery and mutual dialogue between teacher and pupil.

Revisionist/instrumentalism

In these utilitarian ideologies, education must be relevant to the economic and social needs of society by producing a skilled workforce. Vocational relevance is a key principle of curricula and the teaching of science and technology is emphasized. Scrimshaw (1983) further subdivides instrumentalism into traditional and adaptive. The former is concerned with the learning of specific vocational skills, whereas the latter aims to equip the learner to be adaptable to the changing needs of society.

Reconstructionism

This ideology sees education as means of bringing about social change through analysis discussion and reconstruction of social issues. The key teaching approach is small-group methods.

The above review of ideologies portrays them as mutually incompatible, but in practice elements of different ideological derivation are often combined to meet the needs of a given curriculum design. For example, curricula for health care professionals are by their very nature instrumental in ideology, in that their purpose is to produce a skilled professional workforce. However, they also reflect a progressive ideology in their emphasis on the personal and professional growth of the individual and by the adoption of such strategies as student–teacher negotiation and learning by experience.

Curriculum theory

The purpose of theory is to try to understand and explain phenomena, and curriculum theory attempts to relate educational scholarship to pragmatic everyday aspects of educational practice. Theories provide a rationale for making decisions about the curriculum and consist of concepts combined together to form statements. Concepts are mental constructs which an individual employs to make sense of the environment, i.e. classes of objects, events or situations that possess common properties. In terms of curriculum theory, the component concepts include pupil/student, teacher, goals, content, methods and evaluation, as well as concepts of coherence and progression. In curriculum theory, the concepts may be combined as association statements, which state that two or more concepts are related, or as causal statements that postulate a cause and effect relationship between the concepts. In curriculum studies, theories are often expressed as models of curriculum, the terms being used interchangeably.

The classic curriculum models

A model is a physical or conceptual representation of something; physical models are replicas of objects, and may be actual size or built to scale. Curriculum models are conceptual models, i.e. simplified representations of reality in graphic, mathematical or symbolic form. Models of curriculum help to clarify thinking about the nature of curriculum and a number of models have become well established within the literature.

Product model or behavioural-objectives model

Although having its origins in certain writings at the turn of the century, this model is usually ascribed to Ralph Tyler. In his book *Basic Principles of Curriculum and Instruction* (Tyler, 1949), he articulated a rationale for effective curriculum, viewing education as 'a process of changing the behaviour patterns of people, using behaviour in the broad sense to include thinking and feeling as well as overt action' (Tyler, 1949, p. 5). He identifies four fundamental questions to be answered in developing a curriculum.

1. What educational purposes should the school seek to attain?
2. How can learning experiences be selected that are likely to be useful in attaining these objectives?
3. How can learning experiences be organized for effective instruction?
4. How can the effectiveness of learning experiences be evaluated? (Tyler, 1949, p. 1).

This notion of rational curriculum planning was taken up by a number of writers and led to the generic model of curriculum as consisting of four main components: objectives, content, method and evaluation. Hence, the emphasis on this model is on the achievement of objectives by the student. In other words, it is an output model. Tyler stressed the importance of stating objectives in terms of student behaviours: 'any statement of the objectives of the school should be a statement of changes to take place in students' (Tyler, 1949, p. 44). This emphasis on student behaviours was taken up by other proponents of the model and led to a move to limit behavioural objectives to observable, measurable changes in behaviour, leaving no room for such things as 'understanding' or 'appreciation'.

This restrictive interpretation of objectives has been the subject of much criticism, as it then becomes difficult to formulate objectives for higher-level outcomes, and it tends to encourage trivialization of learning by focusing on lower-level outcomes. Opponents of the model claim that it is unsuitable for science subjects, as it emphasizes the learning of factual information rather than scientific enquiry, and that its use encourages conformity rather than diversity.

In an attempt to avoid this dogmatic interpretation of behavioural objectives, some educators have adopted a learning outcomes approach in their curricula. Learning outcomes, while being statements of direction, are couched in much more general terms than behavioural objectives, as shown in the examples below.

1. Explore the meaning and underlying philosophy of health promotion.
2. Develop an understanding of basic statistical concepts in relation to research design and be able to apply these as appropriate.

The objectives model offers a rational design process that can be used regardless of the underlying educational ideology of the curriculum.

Stenhouse's process model

The objectives model described above sets out a rational process for designing curricula, but the term 'process' is used in quite a different sense to describe models which emphasize the process of education – i.e. the learning experiences of students – rather than the product – i.e. the behavioural outcomes of instruction.

Lawrence Stenhouse was a major critic of the objectives model of curriculum. He saw the use of behavioural objectives as acting as a filter that distorted knowledge in schools.

The filtering of knowledge through an analysis of objectives gives the school an authority and power over its students by setting arbitrary limits to speculation and by defining arbitrary solutions to unresolved problems of knowledge. This translates the teacher from the role of the student of a complex field of knowledge to the role of the master of the school's agreed version of that field. (Stenhouse, 1975, p. 86)

He stated that the minimum requirements for a curriculum are that it should offer:

A. in planning:
1. principles for the selection of content: what is to be learned and taught;
2. principles for the development of a teaching strategy: how it is to be learned and taught;
3. principles for the making of decisions about sequence;
4. principles on which to diagnose the strengths and weaknesses of individual students and differentiate the general principles 1, 2 and 3 above. to meet individual cases;

B. in empirical study:
1. principles on which to study and evaluate the progress of students;
2. principles on which to study and evaluate the progress of teachers;
3. guidance as to the feasibility of implementing the curriculum in varying school contexts, pupil contexts, environments and peer-group situations;
4. information about the variability of effects in differing contexts and on different pupils and an understanding of the causes of the variation;

C. in relation to justification:
a formulation of the intention or aim of the curriculum which is accessible to critical scrutiny.

Stenhouse believed that it was possible to organize the curriculum without having to specify in advance the behavioural changes that should occur in students; indeed, he argued that the purpose of education was to make student outcomes unpredictable. Knowledge does not consist of 'known facts' to be remembered, rather, it provides a basis for speculation and conjecture about a discipline.

The content of a curriculum can be selected on the basis that it is worthwhile in itself and not merely as the means to achievement of a behavioural objective. Stenhouse uses the term 'principles of procedure' for statements of worthwhileness, and for teaching these are couched in terms of what the teacher will do rather than what the students will be able to do – for example, 'to encourage students to reflect on their experiences'.

The role of assessment in a process curriculum is very different from that in a product model, being that of critic rather than marker. The teacher is cast in the role of critical appraiser of the student's work, with the emphasis on developing self-appraisal in the student. 'The worthwhile activity in which teacher and student are engaged has standards and criteria immanent in it and the task of appraisal is that of improving students' capacity to work to such criteria by critical reaction to work done. In this sense, assessment is about the teaching of self-assessment' (Stenhouse, 1975, p. 95).

Stenhouse's approach reflects the romantic/progressivism ideologies of children's education, but his emphasis on the process of education has created interest within health care education curricula.

Lawton's cultural-analysis model

This model was developed by Denis Lawton as a reaction against what he sees as the dangers of the behavioural objectives model. As the name implies, this model proposes a curriculum planned on the technique of cultural analysis. Culture is defined as the whole way of life of a society and the purpose of education is 'to make available to the next generation what we regard as the most important aspects of culture' (Lawton, 1983). Cultural analysis is the process by which a selection is made from the culture and, in terms of curriculum-planning, Lawton suggests that cultural analysis will ask the following questions.

1. What kind of society already exists?
2. In what ways is it developing?
3. How do its members appear to want it to develop?
4. What kinds of values and principles will be involved in deciding on 3, and on the educational means of achieving 3?

Lawton offers a five-stage model for this analysis.

Stage 1. Cultural invariants. This examines all the aspects that human societies have in common, such as economic and moral aspects, beliefs and other systems.

Stage 2. Cultural variables. Involves analysing the differences between cultures in each of the systems.

Stage 3. Selection from the culture. This stage consists of comparing the cultural analysis of the systems with the existing school curriculum.

Stage 4. Psychological questions and theories. This stage is not in direct continuity with the previous stages, but is seen as an important consideration for any curriculum development.

Stage 5. Curriculum organization. In this final stage the curriculum can now be planned on the basis of the cultural analysis carried out in the previous stages, bearing in mind the important psychological questions and theories that influence learning and instruction.

Lawton's model of curriculum attempts to apply a rational system of analysis to the problem of curriculum content; it is designed for the school curriculum for children and approaches the task of curriculum-planning in a broader way. As Lawton points out in his preface 'the problems of young people growing up in a complex urban, industrialized society have been seriously underestimated; schools have generally failed to take seriously the moral, social and political aspects of culture in relation to curriculum planning' (Lawton, 1983). Lawton's emphasis on the transmission of culture reflects the conservative/classical humanism ideologies of children's education.

Beattie's fourfold model of curriculum

As stated earlier in this chapter, Beattie draws upon the work of Skilbeck (1984) in his 'fourfold model of the curriculum' (Beattie, 1987). Drawing upon his experience with nursing curricula, he suggests that there are four fundamental approaches to the task of planning a curriculum for nursing, each with its own particular strengths and weaknesses.

1. **The curriculum as a map of key subjects:** As the name implies, this approach consists of mapping out the key subjects in the nursing curriculum, preferably integrating them by means of themes such as 'the human life-span' to avoid the danger of an isolated collection of topics.
2. **The curriculum as a schedule of basic skills.** This approach emphasizes the explicit specification of basic skills of nursing, these skills being culled from recent empirical research into nursing practice. A behavioural objectives approach can be appropriate here, provided that it is not used dogmatically for all aspects of teaching, particularly in relation to the knowledge base for clinical practice.
3. **The curriculum as a portfolio of meaningful personal experiences.** This approach puts the student at the centre of things by organizing the curriculum around their interests and experiences. This is done by using a variety of experiential techniques such as action-research, critical incidents, role-play and the like. There will always be a degree of tension between the unpredictability consequent upon student autonomy and the need to ensure sufficient opportunity to cover key areas.
4. **The curriculum as an agenda of important cultural issues.** This approach avoids giving detailed subject matter, focusing instead on controversial issues and political dilemmas in nursing and health care.

These issues are chosen because they are open to debate and have no right answer, thereby stimulating discussion and enquiry.

Beattie suggests that there are three ways of combining the fourfold framework. The first one he calls the 'eclectic curriculum', in which the four approaches are mixed together in some sort of combination. The main problem with this is that the more traditional approaches tend to dominate, leaving only the marginal inclusion of student-centred ideas. Another way is to negotiate each of the key areas with the consumers, the 'negotiated curriculum'.

The third way Beattie calls the 'dialectical curriculum', in which the curriculum designer 'goes out to do battle', as it were, to engage in a deliberate, principled and committed struggle to combat, challenge and contest the dominant codes of curriculum (Beattie, 1987, p. 31). In his 'fourfold model of curriculum' Beattie argues that 'curriculum planners in nursing can and must move beyond simple-minded, "single-model" approaches and towards complex, multifaceted strategies' (Beattie, 1987, p. 32).

Beattie's model is interesting in that it draws upon elements of all five educational ideologies described earlier in the chapter. In fact, his approach is not so much a model as a pragmatic and insightful design specification from which specific nursing curricula can be developed.

Curriculum models derived from learning theorists

The foregoing models of curriculum were largely developed for the education of children, but have been adapted by health care educators to provide a rationale for their curriculum decisions. There are, however, other models, which have had a profound influence on curriculum planning in health care education but which were not designed primarily as curriculum models. These models are designed by learning theorists and their focus is the nature and process of human learning, but they inevitably overlap into the realm of curriculum because they serve as models of how to organize health care education for the most effective learning to take place. Although often linked to ideological stances, some of these models can to some extent be seen as less value-laden and more preoccupied with the means by which learning is achieved – an important consideration in any education and training situation. Because they tend to put the student at the centre of the learning process, these models have greater relevance to health care education; indeed, it could be argued that the use of these as curriculum models is an indication of the inadequacy of the orthodox, school-derived paradigm. They could be seen as interim models of curriculum that fall somewhere between the orthodox and the newly emerging paradigms of health care education, or alternatively as models that transcend the two paradigms.

 Knowles's andragogical model

Malcolm S. Knowles focuses on adult learning and has developed a system called andragogy, which he regards as a new approach to learning in contrast to the traditional model of pedagogy.

The term 'pedagogy' is defined as the art and science of teaching children and is contrasted with 'andragogy', the art and science of 'teaching adults', although the word literally means teaching men. These two models of learning are seen as parallel, not in opposition and Knowles acknowledges that both are appropriate, depending upon circumstances. The two models operate on different assumptions about the learner on five dimensions.

1. **The concept of the learner:** Pedagogy emphasizes dependence and teacher control; andragogy values self-direction and responsibility.
2. **The role of the learner's experience:** Pedagogy makes little use of children's experience; andragogy acknowledges the richness and diversity of adult experience as a basis for learning.
3. **The learner's readiness to learn:** Children's readiness to learn is dependent upon biological maturation and school level; adult readiness is needs-related.
4. **The learner's orientation to learning:** Pedagogy adopts a subject-centred approach to curriculum; andragogy a life-centred, problem-solving approach.
5. **Motivation to learn:** In a pedagogical approach, external motivation by teachers and parents predominates; andragogy values internal motivation to succeed.

Both pedagogy and andragogy may be appropriate models for children and adults; it might be that a pedagogical model would be appropriate when the learner first encounters new or unusual learning situations. Knowles believes that andragogy will be appropriate for children and suggests that many of the facets of pedagogy are the result of a conditioning process by schools.

The implementation of the andragogical model involves a 'process design' as opposed to the pedagogical one of a 'content plan'. The process design consists of seven elements (Knowles, 1984).

1. **Setting the climate for learning.** This involves both the physical and the psychological climate; the former takes account of the seating arrangements and decor and the latter of such things as mutual respect, collaboration, mutual trust and supportiveness, openness and authenticity and a climate of pleasure and humaneness.
2. **Involving learners in mutual planning.** This can be achieved by inviting members to serve on the planning committee and to state their preferences.
3. **Involving learners in the diagnosis of their learning needs.** There is often tension between the needs of participants and the needs of the organization, so these must be negotiated with care. Knowles favours a competency-based model.
4. **Involving learners in the formulation of their objectives.** This can be done by using learning contracts that the learner negotiates.
5. **Involving learners in the design of learning plans.** This is also part of the learning contract, as is the next element.
6. **Helping learners to carry out their learning plans.**
7. **Involving learners in evaluating their learning.** This should include qualitative as well as quantitative evaluation.

Knowles's model reflects the romantic/progressivism ideology and his approach has been widely adopted in curricula for health care education. Its appeal lies in its central tenet, the empowerment of the student, who is highly autonomous and a major partner in the entire curriculum process, from goal-setting to assessment. Knowles's process design for andragogy does not, however, encompass the needs of the employer in the health care sector. In the new context of contracting for education, the latter is assuming paramount importance, and this has major implications for Knowles's process design.

Rogers's humanistic model

Carl Rogers pioneered the concept of client-centred therapy as an alternative to Freudian psychoanalysis. He turned his attention to education and formulated a student-centred approach to learning (Rogers, 1969) which is encapsulated in his principles of learning. These are as follows.

1. Human beings have a natural potentiality for learning.
2. Significant learning takes place when the subject matter is perceived by the student as having relevance for his own purposes.
3. Learning that involves a change in self-organization is threatening and tends to be resisted.
4. Those elements of learning that are threatening to the self are more easily perceived and assimilated when external threats are at a minimum.
5. When threat to the self is low, experience can be perceived in differentiated fashion, and learning can proceed.
6. Much significant learning is acquired through doing.
7. Learning is facilitated when the student participates responsibly in the learning process.
8. Self-initiated learning, which involves the whole person of the learner – feelings as well as intellect – is the most lasting and pervasive.
9. Independence, creativity and self-reliance are all facilitated when self-criticism and self-evaluation are basic and evaluation by others is of secondary importance.
10. The most socially useful learning in the modern world is the learning of the process of learning, a continuing openness to experience and incorporation into oneself of the process of change.

These 10 principles illustrate Rogers's approach to learning and his emphasis on relevance, student participation and involvement, self-evaluation and the absence of threat in the classroom. Rogers sees the teacher as a facilitator of learning: a provider of resources for learning and someone who shares her/his feelings as well as her/his knowledge with the students. Thus the prerequisites of an effective facilitator of learning are awareness of self, being oneself in the classroom, acceptance and trust of the students and understanding and empathy.

Rogers has further articulated his approach to education (Rogers, 1983), seeing learning as a continuum with much meaningless material at one end and significant or experiential learning at the other. The latter has a number of characteristics such as personal involvement, self-initiation, pervasiveness, self-evaluation and meaningfulness. He contrasts the kind of learning that is concerned solely with cognitive functioning with that involving the whole person. Teaching, according to Rogers, is a highly overrated activity, in contrast to the notion of facilitation. Teaching by giving knowledge does not meet the requirements of today's changing world; what is required is the facilitation of learning and change and this calls for a different set of qualities in the facilitator.

The most important factor is the relationship that exists between facilitator and learner and Rogers suggests a number of qualities that are required for this:

1. **Genuineness**, i.e. the facilitator comes across as a real person rather than as some kind of ideal model; hence it is important that s/he shows normal reactions to the students so that they accept her/him as a real person;
2. **Trust and acceptance**, i.e. acceptance of the student as a person in her/his own right as a person who is worthy of respect and care;
3. **Empathic understanding**, i.e. putting oneself in the student's shoes in order to see and understand things from her/his perspective.

Rogers suggests that it is possible for the teacher to build into a programme the freedom to learn, which students require. This can be done by using students' own experiences and problems so that relevance is obvious and by providing resources for the students in the form of both material and human resources.

He also recommends the use of learning contracts that help to give the students autonomy over their own learning. The goal of education is for the student to become a fully functioning person.

The Rogersian approach to education has had great influence on health care curricula, sharing similar values to those espoused for patient/client care, such as independence, self-reliance and active participation in the process of care. The approach reflects very much a romantic/progressive ideology, with its emphasis on personal growth and experiential learning, and also the democratic/liberal humanist ideology of relevance and lifelong learning. Rogers's model transfers very well to the education of health care professionals and his 10 principles of learning remain largely relevant in this context. However, it does tend to go overboard on experiential learning, leaving little place for more formal types of teaching. In the new context of contracting for education, the effective use of resources becomes a major consideration, begging the question of how experiential learning can be managed entirely on an individual student basis, even if this was desirable educationally.

Kolb's experiential learning cycle

Kolb focuses on the nature of learning from experience, and has described an experiential learning cycle (Kolb, 1984). The cycle begins with some kind of concrete experience, professional or personal, that the individual considers interesting or problematic. Observations and information are gathered about the experience and then s/he reflects upon it, replaying it over again and analysing it until certain insights begin to emerge in the shape of a 'theory' about the experience. The implications arising from this conceptualization can then be used to modify existing practice or to generate new approaches to it.

There are four generic adaptive abilities that are required for effective learning:

1. **Concrete experience (CE)**. The student must immerse herself fully and openly in new experiences;
2. **Reflective observation (RO)**. The student must observe and reflect on concrete experiences from a variety of perspectives;
3. **Abstract conceptualization (AC)**. The student must create concepts that integrate her observations into logical theories;
4. **Active experimentation**. The student must apply these theories in decision-making and problem-solving.

Kolb's model has been used extensively within further and higher education, particularly in the areas of vocational and professional education. It has general applicability to any practice-based or work-based education and training, and offers a rationale for the accreditation of prior experiential learning.

DESTABILIZING THE ORTHODOX PARADIGM

Health care education curricula have tended to adopt relatively uncritically the models and ideologies of the school-focused paradigm. Of course, models have been described which purport to be centred on the needs of health care professionals, but in reality these are merely superficial adaptations of existing models that pay scant regard to the specific context of the health professional. This becomes a potentially fatal weakness in the changing context of health care education described below.

In Table 1.1 the main features of the orthodox paradigm were identified. It is rooted in the education of children and its basic constructs have changed little over the years. In this paradigm, the teachers are seen as the prime movers of curriculum design; the range of ideologies and models provide a menu from which they select those that are closest to their beliefs and values about education, and these in turn serve as the philosophical underpinnings of the curriculum design. Health care educators do consult with employers, but the nature of such consultation differs between the two paradigms. The inadequacy of the orthodox paradigm is most tellingly revealed by the superficiality of attempts to match employer needs within curriculum design. Even orthodox instrumentalism as normally applied leaves educators with at least a partial information vacuum with regard to employer needs. Typically employer groups act as advisors to course teams for whom their advice takes a low priority compared with institutionalized 'professional' or 'educational' priorities of the sort described in the above review. This contrasts markedly with the corporate paradigm, where the employer's workforce supply needs become the most important factor in curriculum design. In this paradigm, the health care educators role is to bring their expertise to bear on the design of curricula that fulfil the requirements of the employer. In these circumstances, attempts to empathize with employers' positions are less superficial (Chapters 8 and 9).

A variety of factors has begun to expose the increasing inadequacy of the orthodox paradigm for health care education, and these are discussed in the following sections.

The winds of change in health care

Over the past 10 years the National Health Service has been subject to constant and relentless change. Health care education, by its very nature, cannot fail to be influenced by the changes occurring within the NHS, but is also affected by changes in the wider field of education. Several key changes that have, or will have, implications for health care education, are identified below.

Professionalization

The training of health care professionals for nursing, midwifery and the professions supplementary to medicine has traditionally taken place in educational institutions within the NHS. The past decade, however, has seen a progressive shift in the location of courses for professions supplementary to medicine into the further and higher education sector, reflecting the aspirations of these professions to redefine their basic training to undergraduate level. In Chapter 3, Alan Walker and John Humphreys discuss this from the point of view of physiotherapy education.

The nursing profession was not immune to this 'upward professional mobility' trend, and the publication of *Project 2000: A New Preparation for Practice* (UKCC, 1986) required that training for registration as a nurse should be to at least Diploma of Higher Education level. This was to be achieved by colleges of nursing and midwifery linking with local institutions of higher education, and these new relationships led in some cases to total incorporation of the former into higher education. This linking with higher education had profound effects on the curriculum, with nurse/midwife teachers having to adapt to the new and often unfamiliar systems and philosophy of the partner institution.

Credit accumulation and transfer schemes (CATS)

Credit accumulation and transfer schemes began to make a real impact upon higher education in the mid-1980s, and most institutions, including the ENB, are now designing their educational provision within a CAT framework. In CAT schemes, a specified number of credit points is awarded to the student on successful completion of appropriate learning. This learning can be gained in three ways: through formal study on a course, from existing qualifications, or by learning gained from professional or life experience.

The CATS system of credit points takes as its standard a three-year full-time undergraduate honours degree course, which is credit rated at 360 credit points, 120 for each of the three years of the course. Each year represents a specific level of learning: First Year = Level 1; Second Year = Level 2; Third Year = Level 3. There is also a Level M for postgraduate study at masters degree level. Credit points gained from appropriate learning can accumulate towards a higher education award such as a diploma or degree, and the amount and level of credit normally required for these is shown in Table 2.1.

Table 2.1 Credit points awarded for appropriate learning

Award	Amount	Level
Certificate	120	1
Diploma	120	2
Bachelors degree	120	3
Postgraduate diploma	70	M
Masters degree	120	M

One of the fundamental principles of CAT schemes is that students who have been awarded credit points from one institution can transfer them to studies in another institution. The contribution of existing credits, gained outside the awarding institution, towards a higher education award is termed accreditation of prior learning (APL).

In order for credit to count towards an award it must be relevant to that award and be at an appropriate level. The length of time since the course was completed also affects its current relevance, so APL is normally confined to courses completed within the previous five years. There is normally a maximum percentage of APL that can be counted towards an award, which may vary between institutions.

Credit awarded to a student for specified learning in one institution is termed **general credit** and can be transferred to studies in other higher education institutions. The receiving institution, however, may decide that only a proportion of this general credit is actually relevant to their curriculum, and this proportion of the general credit is termed specific credit. If any specific credit matches the learning outcomes of a unit on the course to which the student is transferring, then s/he can be given exemption from that unit.

Prior learning can be gained not only from attendance at courses, but also learning gained from the day-to-day experience of professional practice or of life generally, as in rearing a child or writing a book. This is termed accreditation of prior experiential learning (APEL). It is important to note that experience alone is insufficient; the student must demonstrate how s/he has learned from the experience. Credit points can be given for such experiential learning provided that it is relevant to the award which the student is seeking to achieve, and that a portfolio of evidence for such learning has been presented for accreditation to the awarding institution.

It is useful at this point to draw a distinction between competence-based APEL and professional-development APEL (Butterworth, 1993). The widest application of the former is in the national vocational qualifications (NVQ) field, where the emphasis is very much on the production of satisfactory evidence of previous performance by the claimant.

In the professional-development type of APEL evidence of past achievements must also be produced by the claimant, but in addition s/he must produce an analysis of that evidence, including its significance to their professional development. This must be supported by relevant theoretical perspectives.

In CATS the term 'scheme' is used to denote the overall framework of regulations that govern the academic awards within the scheme. These awards are the higher education qualifications such as diplomas and degrees referred to above. Within an institution's CAT scheme there will be a number of pathways leading to academic awards. The term 'pathway' is used instead of 'course' since the latter implies a relatively fixed, linear sequence of content. A pathway consists of many units (also termed modules in some institutions) from which the student can negotiate a programme of study to suit their individual professional and personal needs. A CAT scheme, therefore, consists of large numbers of units that are potentially available to the student. The individual pathway regulations will distinguish between units that are compulsory or core, and those that are options.

Normally units can be done in any order within a pathway, although some units may be designated as prerequisites for other units according to the nature of the pathway. Units are free-standing and self-contained, with assessment linked to learning outcomes.

CATS has made an enormous impact on the design of health care curricula, exploding as it does many of the 'sacred cows' of curriculum theory. In the past, the coherence of a course was defined by the curriculum planners via their choice of subject matter for inclusion within the course. Similarly, progression was built into the course by the linear sequence of subject matter. Suddenly, the planners are faced with the task of finding new ways to define coherence and progression, with establishing systems for evaluating students' prior learning, and with setting up management structures to deal with the complexity of CAT schemes. Putting the student in the 'driving seat' has major implications for the role of the teacher, in that the relationship becomes a partnership. The student is given the responsibility for determining coherence and progression, by matching the choice of study units to her/his own professional role and needs.

Val Thompson and Dai Hall discuss a credit scheme for nurses and midwives developed by the Princess Alexandra and Newham College of Nursing and Midwifery, in partnership with the University of Greenwich, in Chapter 3.

Open learning

Open learning is a flexible approach to learning that is characteristically learner-centred and which uses multimedia learning materials, tutorial guidance and support (Quinn, 1988). The notion of 'openness' is a relative one, given that educational programmes will vary widely in the degree of control that students have over their learning. This control encompasses the whole spectrum of learning, including the aims and objectives, content, teaching and learning methods and assessment, as well as the question of access to courses and pattern or mode of study.

Open learning attempts to remove any barriers that prevent an individual from gaining access to education or training, by offering flexible provision that takes into account the individual's needs and learning style. Many health professionals find it extremely difficult to undertake continuing professional education; health authorities have been unable or unwilling to pay fees and expenses for further professional study, and have found it difficult to release staff for study leave with the result that they have to pursue studies in their own time while holding down a full-time job. There are also those professionals bringing up young families and whose commitments preclude attendance at an educational institution; open learning offers such professionals the opportunity to continue their education.

Working for patients: Working Paper 10

The government's Working Paper 10 (Department of Health, 1989) has ushered in a new approach to educational provision, with a competitive training environment being introduced through a system of contracting for education. Colleges of nursing are no longer automatically funded to provide courses at pre- and post-registration levels, but instead are required to bid for educational contracts with service providers, via regional health authorities.

Service providers have become clients of the colleges of nursing, and as such will require these colleges to provide education and training that meets identified staff development needs. This has necessitated a shift in orientation from a teacher-led to a client-centred approach to educational provision, and if colleges cannot meet the requirements of the service providers, contracts will not be awarded. Contracting for education is a means of ensuring that service providers obtain the kind of education and training that best suits their staff development needs. Instead of being invited to send staff on courses that the college already has on offer, the service providers will be able to state precisely their specific education and training requirements. They will also be able to monitor the quality of the educational provision and provide feedback on college performance. In turn, the colleges will have to adopt a client-centred approach to curriculum design and delivery, and teaching staff may have difficulty initially in accepting the shift in control from themselves to the service providers. They may also be anxious about the competitive contracting process, and what might happen if they fail to win contracts.

The special nature of health care professional education

Allowing for the fact that established educational ideologies refer to the education of children, it could be said that professional education reflects utilitarian revisionist/instrumentalism ideologies, since its primary purpose is the preparation of professional practitioners.

While acknowledging that professional education may also develop the individual, this is not its primary purpose; rather, it is the means to an end. Concepts such as the 'rounded person' and 'liberal studies' are evident in many professional curricula, and beg the question why employers should have to pay for something which may be already taught in compulsory schooling. It is useful at this stage to distinguish between compulsory education, i.e. education to age 16 in the schools sector, and post-compulsory education, i.e. voluntary education in schools, colleges and universities. The aims of compulsory education are reflected in the educational ideology underpinning any given curriculum, but broadly speaking they have been of a general nature, for example, studies for the General Certificate of Secondary Education (GCSE). This general nature of compulsory education is now giving way to a much more vocational orientation, as exemplified by the emergence of the new General National Vocational Qualifications (GNVQs). These are termed the new 'vocational A Levels', but are also offered at Foundation and Intermediate levels which equate to four or five GCSEs at grades D–G and A–C respectively.

Post-compulsory education can be said to be largely specific in its aims and focus, whether these be academic, vocational or professional (Squires, 1987). There is no clear distinction between these, however; academic education is synonymous with higher education, but much professional education also takes place in universities; vocational education, often referred to as further education, is about preparation for work, but so is professional education.

The most commonly perceived difference between vocational and professional education is the greater knowledge base and role autonomy required for professional practice; this distinction is often referred to as training versus education. Training is usually categorized as the learning of performance skills, with little or no reference to any underlying knowledge base. Education, on the other hand, is seen as the development of a comprehensive knowledge base and a repertoire of cognitive skills such as problem-solving and critical thinking. This unhelpful dichotomy leads inevitably to the denigration of training in comparison with education, relegating it to the repetitive performance of basic tasks that require no thought or understanding.

In reality, however, most occupations involve elements of both theory and practice, so it is better to conceptualize education and training as being at the opposite ends of a continuum. Health professional education, with its emphasis on both theory and practice, would fall midway between the poles, whereas that of a health care support worker would be closer to the training end of the continuum. A useful classification is that made in the Haslegrave Report (BTEC, 1987), which identifies three occupational levels, professional, technician and craftsman. The highest level is the professional, and the lowest level the craftsman.

The technician level falls midway between the other two, and is characterized by an understanding of the general principles and purposes of the work. Unlike craftsmen or operatives, who rely on established practices and skills, the technician is able to exercise technical judgements about the work.

The work of Donald Schon makes a useful contribution to the debate about professional education, offering insight into the nature of professional knowledge and how it differs from academic, scientific knowledge (Schon, 1991). He maintains that professional practice involves the use of tacit, intuitive knowledge; the professional practitioner has the ability to reflect upon this knowledge whilst s/he is engaged in the activities of practice, and this enables her/him to deal with unique, unpredictable or conflicting situations. This notion of the reflective practitioner, according to Schon, contrasts markedly with the prevailing model of professional practice, the technical rationality model.

Technical rationality views professional practice as the application of general, standardized, theoretical principles to the solving of practice problems. This top-down view puts general theoretical principles at the top of the hierarchy of professional knowledge and practical problem-solving at the bottom, leading to current situation in education, i.e. the pre-eminence of theory and the denigration of practice. Schon cites the position of research in relation to practice, with the former conducted in different institutions to those in which the profession is practised. He also notes that research is seen as more prestigious that practice, and we can draw a parallel between this point and the fact that professional educators are seen as more prestigious by the practitioners themselves.

Technical rationality, therefore, views professional practice as a process of instrumental problem-solving, with the assumption that problems are self-evident. Schon, however, argues that in reality practitioners are not presented with problems *per se*, but with problem-situations. These must be converted into actual problems by a process of problem-setting, i.e. selecting the elements of the situation, deciding the ends and means and framing the context. According to Schon, the reflective practitioner is characterized by a range of personal qualities and abilities, such as the ability to engage in self-assessment; to criticize the existing state of affairs; to promote change and to adapt to change; and to practise as an autonomous professional. He also distinguishes between the effective and the ineffective practitioner: the former is able to recognize and explore confusing or unique events that occur during practice, whereas the latter is confined to repetitive and routine practice, neglecting opportunities to think about what s/he is doing.

THE DEMISE OF CURRICULUM

The foregoing sections of this chapter have argued that the orthodox, school-derived paradigm has been destabilized by a variety of factors, and is no longer legitimate as a rational basis for the design of health care education.

The orthodox paradigm encouraged educators to follow a linear progression from ideology to curriculum, and led to a belief that educators knew best what the curriculum should be. Ironically, this model is more that of a technician than a professional, since the hallmark of a professional is the concept of partnership with a client. A proper college–employer relationship is more demanding and rewarding than the existing system, in that the teachers must become professional educators in a similar way to other professionals who function on the basis of trust between themselves and their clients. However, it is important at this point to distinguish who is the client of the college. The primary client of the professional educator, and thus of the college, is the NHS employer and the secondary clients are the students.

I am very much aware that this interpretation omits any mention of the patient as a client. I would argue strongly, however, that it is not the responsibility of the college to provide patient care, rather, it is to provide education and training that meets the employer's requirements, since patient care is their responsibility. In fact, by arguing that the patient is the client of the educators, the college can avoid the necessity of engaging the employer in dialogue about the educational requirements of the service, and this attitude goes some way towards explaining the education–service (theory–practice) gap that has for so long been a source of conflict at the heart of the health care education system. The gap is the result of the different expectations of the profession and the employer. The profession's main concern is the training of a registered practitioner in accordance with its criteria, whereas the employer requires a staff nurse who can function effectively as part of the workforce. While these expectations can and should be the same, in reality the profession seems to view the three-year training programme as only the first stage in the production of a qualified practitioner. Hence, recently qualified staff nurses are encouraged to undertake further training by means of Staff Nurse Development Programmes. Employers might legitimately question why, after three years of education and training, the staff nurse is not fully equipped to undertake her role in the workforce without undertaking yet more training soon after qualifying.

Within the field of health care practice, great store is set upon the relationships between practitioner and patient/client. Similarly, within the health care education setting the teacher–student relationship occupies a pre-eminent position. It is interesting, therefore, to examine college–employer relationships and to attempt to draw comparisons between these and the relationships mentioned above. The former are characterized by mutual trust, respect, empathy and willingness to work together for the benefit of the patient or student. However, college–employer relationships seem to be characterized by quite the reverse sentiments, in that there is mutual distrust, little respect for each other's expertise, even less empathy for each other, and often overt antagonism between the parties. It is important to ask why this particular relationship should be so different from the other two.

I maintain that service providers, like patients and students, are individuals with rights, and that professional educators have a responsibility towards them.

This responsibility should aim to marry up the needs of the individual professional employee with those of the organization, resolving conflicts as appropriate. They must have sympathy with employers' needs, and can help by engaging in dialogue with them. In addition, curriculum evaluation must include the needs of the employer/client as the major aspect. Hence, the characteristics of the prevailing curriculum paradigm make it, in my opinion, inappropriate for the newly emerging needs of health care curricula. What is emerging is a new paradigm for health care professional education that is free from the tyranny of the school-focused curriculum paradigm and which acknowledges the reality of health care professional practice in today's climate.

The next three chapters consist of case studies which describe curriculum innovations in three different contexts: nursing, physiotherapy and teacher-training. These case studies are not simply examples of innovative educational practice: they also provide evidence of the new demands not easily addressed within the orthodox paradigm of health care education, and of the ways in which institutions have responded to these.

In the application of credit systems to a professional education and training in which employer needs are a pre-eminent influence, much of the established cannon of orthodox curriculum theory is redundant. Whereas it may still for the time being be a legitimate and useful basis for practice in school age or academic higher education, in health care education 'curriculum' in the orthodox sense is in decline. Whereas the word may remain useful, the old concept and much of its panoply of supporting theory is no longer relevant in a sector increasingly unique in funding and control terms (Chapter 6). It seems likely that the next few years will see the final demise of the orthodox curriculum.

REFERENCES

Beattie, A. (1987) Making a curriculum work, in *The Curriculum in Nursing Education*, (ed. P. Allan and M. Jolley), Croom Helm, London.

Bell, R. (1973) *Thinking About the Curriculum*, Open University Press, Milton Keynes.

BTEC (Business and Technician Education Council) (1987) *BTEC Teachers Guide*, BTEC, London.

Butterworth, C. (1992) More than one bite at the APEL – contrasting models of accrediting prior learning. *Journal of Further and Higher Education*, **16**(3).

Davies, I. (1969) Education and social science. *New Society*, **8 May**.

Department of Health (1989) *Working for Patients, Education and Training*, Working Paper 10, HMSO, London.

Kerr, J. (1968) Changing the curriculum, in *The Curriculum: Design, Context and Development*, (ed. R. Hooper), Oliver & Boyd, Edinburgh.

Knowles, M. (1984) *Andragogy in Action*, Jossey Bass, San Francisco.

Kolb, D.A. (1984) *Experiential Learning: Experience as the Source of Learning and Development*, Prentice Hall, London.

Lawton, D. (1983) *Curriculum Studies and Educational Planning*, Hodder & Stoughton, London.

Lewis, A. and Miel, A. (1972) *Supervision for Improved Instruction: New Challenges, New Responses*, Wadsworth, Belmont.

Quinn, F. (1988) *The Principles and Practice of Nurse Education*, 2nd edn, Chapman & Hall, London.

Rogers, C. (1969) *Freedom to Learn*, Merrill, Ohio.

Rogers, C. (1983) *Freedom to Learn for the 80s*, Merrill, Ohio.

Saylor, J., Alexander, W. and Lewis, A. (1981) *Curriculum Planning for Better Teaching and Learning*, 4th edn, Holt, Rinehart & Winston, New York.

Schon, D.A. (1991) *The Reflective Practitioner: How Professionals Think in Action*, Avebury, Aldershot.

Scrimshaw, P. (1983) *Educational Ideologies*. Unit 2 of Educational Studies, Open University, Milton Keynes.

Skilbeck, M. (1984) *School Based Curriculum Development*, Harper & Row, London.

Squires, G. (1987) *The Curriculum Beyond School*, Hodder & Stoughton, London.

Stenhouse, L. (1975) *An Introduction to Curriculum Research and Development*, Heinemann, London.

Tanner, D. and Tanner, L. (1980) *Curriculum Development: Theory into Practice*, 2nd edn, Macmillan, New York.

Tyler, R. (1949) *Basic Principles of Curriculum and Instruction*, University of Chicago Press, Chicago.

UKCC (United Kingdom Central Council for Nursing, Midwifery and Health Visiting) (1986) *Project 2000: A New Preparation for Practice*, UKCC, London.

3	# Case study: a credit scheme for nurses and midwives

Val Thomson and Dai Hall

Editors' introduction

The focus of this first case study is the joint development of a credit scheme for nursing and midwifery awards between the University of Greenwich and the Princess Alexandra and Newham College of Nursing and Midwifery. The chapter exposes the shortcomings of the orthodox educational paradigm in accommodating a flexible, work-focused approach to learning and describes the development of an innovative credit accumulation and transfer (CAT) scheme that includes the first ENB Higher Award pathway to become operational in England.

THE CHALLENGE TO NURSING AND MIDWIFERY EDUCATION

In August 1989 the UKCC, the statutory body for nurses, midwives and health visitors charged with maintaining and improving standards of education and practice, launched a major project on post-registration education and practice (PREP) (UKCC, 1990). The project report stated that changes in the patterns of health and disease; together with changing institutional arrangements, which include new styles of clinical management, etc., require a concomitant change in the nature of post-registration education and practice. Recognition was given to the effect on education provision of the new ethos of purchaser and providers as the use of contracts is extended to the provision of education.

With rationalization of workforce requirement, investment in highly skilled practitioners must ensure that their individual contribution is maximized and the match between person, their development and their role made as near perfect as possible. In order to do this a radical re-evaluation of current learning patterns was proposed which encompasses the idea of 'upwards and onwards' rather than 'more of the same'. The report called for the introduction of a logical and comprehensive framework for education, based on the principles of credit accumulation and transfer, which would enable practitioners to claim credit for demonstrating learning through existing qualifications or through experiences relating to their area of practice.

Simultaneously, the English National Board for Nursing, Midwifery and Health Visiting (ENB) commissioned a number of related research studies as part of a training needs analysis project which examined these needs in nurses, midwives and health visitors. The studies concluded that continuing education should:

1. link effective continuing education to maintaining and improving the quality of care through an ongoing performance review system;
2. relate quality in continuing education to improved care provided in response to changing client needs and expectations;
3. ensure value for money in continuing education by integrating and consolidating what is already provided;
4. meet the workforce and skill needs of new health care structures through planned professional development;
5. prepare practitioners to make maximum contribution to the reformed health services;
6. contribute to the work of the Board and service by ensuring the right numbers of appropriately prepared practitioners are available to meet the changing health care needs;
7. lead to the qualification of the ENB Higher Award which gives recognition to what has already been accomplished and eradicates any possibility for repetitious learning and training (ENB Framework – Guide to implementation, 1991).

THE CHALLENGE TO HIGHER EDUCATION

In May 1990 the South East England Consortium for Credit Accumulation and Transfer (SEEC) Conference on 'CATS in Practice' was addressed by Norbert Singer, Director of Thames Polytechnic (now the University of Greenwich). In his address Singer described the British higher education system as (generally) elitist and inappropriate because: a) the great majority of the population ended their education at a very early age; b) there are few connections between any professional development people achieve in their careers and the institutions of higher education; c) higher education is traditionally very prescriptive of the learning that people must undergo in order to achieve awards – the learning is institution- rather than individual-focused.

Singer went on to argue that what was needed (if Britain was to remain a key industrial/commercial power) was a higher education system that: a) was open to far more people; b) allowed for the updating of knowledge and skills; c) continued throughout life; and d) allowed people to 'attend' in a variety of modes, inter-mittently and when it suited them. Singer suggested that these needs could be met through a system of higher awards that allowed for credit to be given for a whole variety of learning experiences both inside and outside the higher educa-tion system. Such a system is that of credit accumulation and transfer (CATS).

Another important contributor to thinking about the education of profession-als has been what Foreman-Peck (1993) calls the drive towards the production of 'enterprise graduates'. This drive began in 1985 with a White Paper on higher education into the 1990s. The aim of the enterprise movement is to produce pro-fessionals who are flexible, responsive and autonomous. Through the judicious use of financial awards to institutions the government has sought to encourage the development of courses that foster these qualities.

Clearly, what is needed is a curriculum which in concept and organization is flexible and learner-centred. It should: a) generate autonomy and professionalism; b) recognize the importance of process knowledge achieved through work-focused learning; c) encourage reflection on and in action; d) be low cost; e) involve its commissioners in planning; and f) respond to service providers' needs. Credit ac-cumulation and transfer schemes can in our view achieve these outcomes.

DEVELOPMENTS IN ACADEMIC THINKING

In recent years much work and thought has been expended in exploration of the nature of professionalism and through that into the meaning of professional learn-ing. The possibility of giving credit for non-institutional learning depends on having a clear idea of what this professional learning is and how it comes about.

A particularly useful view of the nature of professional thinking is that of Schon (1983). He has argued that a traditional view of professional processes based on 'technical reality' overstresses the importance of 'the application of scientific theory and technique' and understresses the role of 'reflection in action'. Schon describes reflection in action as a process by which a professional who encounters something unusual in their practice detaches from it for a while and reflects on it. Professional development is a process of constantly reassess-ing and adjusting understanding in the light of such reflection, what Schon calls 'a reflective conversation with the situation'.

Schon explores this notion in considerable depth, making use of many exam-ples from a variety of professions and practices. He uses this theory to place conventional knowledge in the role of underpinning practice and develops the notion of the 'reflective practitioner'. The reflective practitioner is one who is able to adapt to new circumstances, is constantly able to grow professionally and is not limited to routine repetitive practice. The key to becoming such a practitioner is to have developed the appropriate skills and personal attributes.

Eraut (1992) builds on the work of Schon and distinguishes a number of kinds of knowledge and processes which contribute to a person becoming a professional.

The essence of his argument is that (what he calls) 'propositional knowledge' (the codified structure of theory and concepts that makes up the traditional higher education syllabus) is merely a part of what professionals need to know. In order for professionals to act, this propositional knowledge needs to be processed in a number of ways. Eraut identifies as particularly important 'process knowledge'. This is, broadly, the sequence of processes through which a professional goes in carrying out her/his business.

Eraut's work has possibly two implications that are important in the present debate. On the one hand it implies that professional qualifications based only on propositional knowledge are an inadequate preparation for a profession. On the other hand it implies that higher education needs to be prepared to acknowledge process knowledge in the granting of awards.

An important component of acquiring process knowledge is reflection. Kremer-Hayon, in 1990, examined the ideas of Schon and applied them particularly to teaching as a profession. She analysed a series of writings that explored reflection in professional thinking and developed a model for developing reflection in teachers. For her there is no doubt that reflection is the key to teacher development. She distinguishes between 'reflection and professional knowledge' on the one hand and 'pedagogical knowledge' on the other. Reflection turns pedagogic knowledge into professional knowledge. The skill of carrying out this reflection is what enables a person to develop as a teacher.

Much work has been done in the area of reflection. Perhaps the most important of this is that associated with David Kolb and is often characterized as 'the Kolb cycle' or 'the experiential learning cycle'. The essence of the model (Kolb and Fry, 1985) is that learning, change and growth occur through a continuous integrated four-step cycle. It begins with an item of experience (concrete experience); the learner then collects observations and information about this experience (observations and reflections). The fruit of these observations are analysed (abstract conceptualization) and the implications of this analysis are used to formulate new ideas, the modification of behaviour or the planning of new experiences (active experimentation). The cycle can now begin again based on experience deriving from the new experimentation.

These ways of conceptualizing professional learning are important in education for three reasons. Firstly, they have implications for teaching methods. They lie at the core of an 'experiential learning theory' espoused very clearly and cogently by Gibbs and the Further Education Unit (1988). The Kolb cycle is used to rationalize a methodology of teaching based on creating opportunities for students to both learn through and learn to apply the Kolb cycle. Gibbs stresses the importance of reflection in the process and recommends strategies for improving learners' reflective skills.

Secondly, they can offer a rationale for professional courses and through this a basis for assessment. One example is Land (1991) who uses it as a rationale for a course of initial teacher education. Land bases the whole methodology of the course on a view of professional learning which places the role of theory as supporting practice and providing the tools with which to analyse and reflect. He sees teachers as learning through the Kolb cycle. He defines learning in terms of 'self development involving action and reflection' and therefore sets reflection on practice as a key requirement of assessment of student performance.

Thirdly, they can be used to provide the basis for the accreditation of prior experiential learning. The Kolb cycle is the rationale used in the APEL counselling process used at the university of Greenwich (Bloor and Butterworth, 1990; Butterworth, 1992).

CREDIT ACCUMULATION AND TRANSFER SCHEMES

The Further Education Staff College (FESC) in 1989 defined credit accumulation as 'processes which enable learners to acquire qualifications over time from a variety of learning/learning opportunities. The programmes need not be continuous, nor include formal attendance at an institution'. They also define credit transfer as 'the acceptance of an award or credit obtained for one purpose ... as credit towards another award'. Higher education in the UK in the 1980s was characterized by considerable growth in interest in the accreditation of in-company training towards awards. A key feature of many of these schemes is the development of a joint arrangement between the commercial organization and the institution of higher education so that work or study undertaken in the workplace can receive accreditation towards a qualification. Dearden (1991) sets out the key concepts for commercial organizations and acknowledges that 'credit rating of in-company development programmes has already been seen as a real benefit and a sound investment by a significant number of employing organizations'.

Jessup (1991), in his book on the emergence of competence-based systems of setting out training, describes a world in which higher education will need to establish structures and methods of transferring learning derived from 'in-company' training and personal learning into degree and other programmes. It seems to him merely a matter of time before this becomes the norm. It is certainly the case, in the areas of teacher education and nurse and midwife education, that non-institutional providers of training are becoming quite assertive in their expectation that their work will receive accreditation. Jessup's assertion is merely the latest in a series of prophecies in this area.

The credit accumulation scheme for in-service teachers at the University of Greenwich (formerly Thames Polytechnic) began in 1988. It is based on the credit accumulation and transfer regulations of the Council for National Academic Awards (CNAA) (1987) which facilitated the development of CATS in CNAA institutions and laid down the ground rules for a national scheme. This was particularly important if the transfer element was to work effectively.

These rules are in operation (more or less) throughout the old Polytechnic sector (now the new Universities) and include a provision for 'admission with advanced standing', now known as the accreditation of prior learning.

BACKGROUND TO THE DEVELOPMENT

The introduction of such a scheme for nursing and midwifery continuing education challenged programme planners to review and restructure existing provision in a way that offered progression and reduced the duplication of learning that was inherent in previous course design. Both content and course organization must more closely reflect the needs of the user. Davies (1990) explains that trends in employment point to more people engaging in career episodes rather than in careers; people may come forward at diverse ages and with diverse experiences and, secondly, may come from a period in work or not in work. The flexible nature of CATS means that not only can the diversity of experience be recognized and given credit, but the programme of study is tailored to individual need and to episodic participation. The traditional view of curriculum design is radically altered in these circumstances because each programme of study is unique to the individual.

Two important issues emerge.

1. How do educationalists articulate the underlying values and beliefs from which the scheme has developed and determine the nature and assessment of diverse learning opportunities?
2. How can a judgement be made about whether the choice of learning opportunities can be said to meet the requirements of a named professional/academic award?

Following Benner (1984), the notion of the progressive stages of professional development that mark the passage from novice to expert provides a helpful structure through which learning can be organized. The model is related to a concept of lifelong learning proposed by Jarvis (1983) and supported by the continuum of practice described by the UKCC in the PREPP proposals (UKCC, 1990). Thus, initial training provides the 'bedrock' from which practitioners will continue to improve their standards of practice. All must show continued development, but some will wish to move on from primary practice to specialist nursing practice or move further, into advanced practice. Curriculum planning must ensure that the transition between the end of initial training and the beginning of continuing education is seamless. It must also describe the characteristics of practice said to be at a specific level to ensure that the notion of progression is evident and can be measured against agreed criteria.

At this point a potential conflict arises between the philosophy of CATS, which places the student/practitioner at the centre of programme planning, and the interests of other stake holders, namely statutory and academic bodies and employers.

Theoretically, students can make up their programme by claiming credit for a multiplicity of previous learning experiences, choose freely from units available and take them in any order. In reality, curriculum planning identifies the parameters within which students make their choice of learning opportunities or claims, and introduces the notion of prerequisite achievement prior to entry into a unit, while individual programme planning demonstrates the partnership between practitioners, educationalists and service managers.

Today's service managers want a planned work force that is supported by the development of specific attributes. Negotiation at contract setting each year identifies these requirements so that the provision for the coming year consists of current units and newly proposed units based on a need's analysis that reflects local, regional, and national initiatives. Thus a range of units of learning is devised that are available to practitioners who are either registered within the CAT scheme or as associate students with an option to register at a later date.

OPERATIONAL DETAILS OF THE SCHEME

Princess Alexandra and Newham College offer a range of awards under the CATS umbrella, e.g. BSc(Hons) Nursing, Midwifery or Sexual Health, ENB Higher Award, DipHE Midwifery leading to registration on part 10 of the UKCC register. The awards are expressed in terms of credit points and levels. The scheme currently operates at levels 1, 2, and 3; each is the normal equivalent of an undergraduate year. The fourth level, Master's (M), is under development.

Students gain awards by accumulating credit points; an honours degree requires the accumulation of 120 credit points for each of the three levels, 360 credits in total. Normally a full-time year of study yields 120 credit points. The currency of the credit point is awarded for learning demonstrated rather than hours or modules undertaken; a principle that has particular significance when awarding credit for prior learning.

The most important aspect of the structure is flexibility, which is in marked contrast to the more rigidly defined characteristics of traditional courses or even modular systems. Like modular systems however, participants select 'pathways' through a range of available units of learning, and in this sense among others the 'course' is not defined by the education provider but by the participant. Even so, the concept of a 'course' still exists within the scheme and is used to describe clusters of units that together make up ENB certificated courses. Content of the course is grouped into meaningful smaller units of learning, which together make up the whole (Figure 3.1).

This design enables the practitioner to identify any parts for which they could claim exemption by virtue of demonstrating prior learning. They may then choose to complete the ENB course in a shorter time or to undertake a different unit in its place. The latter option also applies to statutorily defined courses such as the DipHE Midwifery leading to registration, where the student may gain credit for prior learning but must still complete the required number of hours of theory and practice.

Each named award is associated with a group of units called a pathway and has its own curriculum philosophy, set of regulations and management structure. The

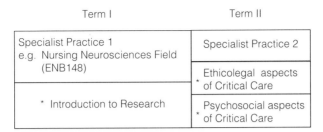

Term I	Term II
Specialist Practice 1 e.g. Nursing Neurosciences Field (ENB148)	Specialist Practice 2
	* Ethicolegal aspects of Critical Care
* Introduction to Research	* Psychosocial aspects of Critical Care

* Units shared by all critical care courses

Figure 3.1 Five units which together make up ENB Critical Care courses.

pathway team is responsible for recruiting and counselling students, teaching and examining the units within its pathway and monitoring quality. Within each pathway, students negotiate their own programme of study, consisting of a package of prior learning and/or units that meet the philosophy and regulations of the pathway and demonstrate progression and coherence for that student.

Each unit is complete (although some units may specify other units as pre-requisites) and is assessed separately. Assessment is based as much as possible on the practice of the student. To facilitate this a proportion of the time a student undertakes to spend on a unit will be spent in her/his own institution. The work that s/he does there will yield the assessment for the unit. Units vary greatly in the kinds of activity they entail: some are based very much in the classroom; others involve work away from the institution such as distance learning, investigations or projects.

A unit could form part of many pathways. For instance, 'HIV and AIDS in babies and young children: a family-centred approach', a unit originally written for the DipHE Midwifery pathway, is also of interest to students undertaking ENB 405 (Special and Intensive Nursing Care of the Newborn) or the BSc in Sexual Health pathway. Shared learning not only encourages the development of shared values and a common culture but also reduces the unit cost by increasing student numbers.

Throughout the scheme, awards, concepts and definitions are expressed in professional terms. There is no distinction between theory and practice; both are subsumed in the notion of professionalism. Some units may emphasize propositional knowledge; some emphasize process knowledge; both are equally important. The relationship between the two is set out in the level definitions.

All levels are clearly defined. Units, assessments and accreditations are judged against these level definitions. Within the University of Greenwich each credit scheme has its own set of level definitions that relate to the nature of learning appropriate for that scheme. An example from our scheme is Level 3: 'Practitioners are specialists within their chosen areas who have developed new professional skills, knowledge and understanding, who have utilized existing research, whose practice is enquiry-based and who promote innovative practice'.

Students enter the scheme at any level if they can demonstrate that they can function at that level. Students can be exempted from Level 1 by virtue of their registration and practice as nurses, midwives and health visitors. Many have gained exemption from Level 2 through a combination of prior certificated and experiential learning, and some have demonstrated considerable work-based learning that meets the outcomes of the ENB Higher Award and can be awarded credit at Level 3.

Throughout the scheme units are written and validated in terms of 'learning outcomes'. The Unit for the Development of Adult Continuing Education (UDACE) report *Learning Outcomes in Higher Education* (Otter, 1992) describes learning outcomes as 'statements of what a learner can do, know and understand as a result of learning'. This is useful as it enables the level of the unit to be established by reference to the level definitions. It also communicates the nature of the unit to potential students and their employers.

Pathway leaders (and through them external examiners) may disallow proposed programmes that fail to demonstrate coherence or contain replication of learning. The parameters of a pathway may be set by designating certain units as core or compulsory, which ensures that the nature of the award is expressed in the choice of units. Students are free to determine the sequence in which they take units, but some units do stipulate prerequisite experience.

The BSc(Hons) Nursing/Midwifery pathway has been designed to reflect the ENB Higher Award characteristics (Table 3.1), which define the role of the practitioner and fall broadly into four main categories: clinical studies, research, management and education. Students must choose a core unit in each of these areas at Level 2; Level 3 choices must include a core unit in clinical studies and the compulsory final research unit. Students who can demonstrate prior learning that meets the outcomes of core units may claim credit and exemption from the unit. The final research unit is synoptic and therefore must be completed. In addition, to achieve the ENB Higher Award the student will show how the 10 key characteristics have been met progressively through the programme of study. S\he must also demonstrate how they have been integrated into practice through the following:

1. a professional portfolio;
2. the research project contained within the research in action unit;
3. a final synoptic assessment.

Within the university each credit scheme has a fixed limit on credit that can be obtained by the demonstration of prior learning. This varies from 50% to 80%. Credit for prior learning can be given for:
1. courses (or parts of courses) done in other institutions;
2. courses provided by employers or other providers;
3. relevant individual experience.

Table 3.1 ENB Summary Card 1: 10 key characteristics

1. Ability to exercise professional accountability and responsibility, reflected in the degree to which the Practitioner uses professional skills, knowledge and expertise in changing environments, across professional boundaries, and in unfamiliar situations.
2. Specialist skills, knowledge and expertise in the practice area where working, including a deeper and broader understanding of client/patient health needs, within the context of changing health care provision.
3. Ability to use research to plan, implement and evaluate concepts and strategies leading to improvements in care.
4. Team working, including multi-professional team working in which the leadership role changes in response to changing client needs, team leadership and team building skills to organize the delivery of care.
5. Ability to develop and use flexible and innovative approaches to practice appropriate to the needs of the client/patient or group in line with the goals of the health service and the employing authority.
6. Understanding and use of health promotion and preventative policies and strategies.
7. Ability to facilitate and assess the professional and other development of all for whom responsible, including where appropriate learners, and to act as a role model of professional practice.
8. Ability to take informed decisions about the allocation of resources for the benefit of individual clients and the client group with whom working.
9. Ability to evaluate quality of care delivered as an ongoing and cumulative process.
10. Ability to facilitate, initiate, manage and evaluate change in practice to improve quality of care.

The definition of levels provides criteria for the judgement of such activities and the award of credit points. Credit can be given for any learning that falls within the definitions whether or not it coincides with a unit offered within a scheme. This contrasts sharply with course-based schemes where admission with advanced standing is almost always limited to exempting applicants from certain elements of the course.

The pathway leader determines how much of the general credit allowable for the above is translated to specific credit allowed against the particular pathway. For instance, a student may wish to claim for child-rearing experience and although this may have relevance for a nursing pathway it might have greater relevance to a midwifery pathway and therefore might be awarded more credit points towards the latter pathway.

The organizational structure of the college continues to be crucial to the development. Princess Alexandra and Newham College (PANC) adopted a matrix management structure that bases its activities on academic theme group membership. Lecturers belong to theme groups and within these plan, teach and assess units specific to the theme. This ensures academic and professional credibility and smooth progression from pre-registration on to post-registration studies. Theme members continue to generate ideas for new units and pathways that reflect their interaction with colleagues in their clinical link area, thereby keeping fingers on the pulse of potential new developments. A good example is the introduction of a Sexual Health pathway, which came about after managers identified a staff development need that was recognized regionally and nationally through the 'Health of the Nation' targets. It was met by the development of a range of related units, providing a specialist but highly marketable route for professional development.

Growth and development within CAT schemes can be rapid. The ethos seems to generate flexibility and responsiveness in staff. The experience within PANC supports this view, and the enthusiasm of the staff has been a major contributory factor to the success of the scheme. The college culture is progressive and encourages creativity. Staff development occurred initially by presentations and then by learning through participation. The CATS strategy group identified and facilitated a number of working groups all feeding back into the strategy group that provided overall direction. Staff were encouraged to join these working groups so that as many people as possible would be involved in the development. As the scheme expands a system of shadowing is employed in which a lecturer observes key activities, then is paired with an experienced lecturer until ready to act alone.

An important aspect of this responsiveness and flexibility is the establishing of a standing committee to validate new units as they are developed. In this way the scheme can respond quickly to the requirements of its clients.

Within the university all schemes share certain key aspects of management. A coordinator/manager is appointed for the scheme as a whole. A Scheme Board is set up which exercises a monitoring and policy-making role. It has places for student representatives. In PANC it includes service managers and policy makers. The Board has at least two major standing subcommittees that carry out key development functions:

1. a Validation Subcommittee which validates all new units developed within the Scheme; this body is chaired by a University representative of the Academic Standards Committee;
2. an Accreditation Subcommittee that is responsible both for the accreditation of courses submitted to the scheme (APL) and for overseeing/monitoring the operation of the APEL process by Pathway Leaders.

The Board, without students and with the additional membership of the external examiners, acts as the assessment board for the scheme as a whole.

Annual reporting is carried out for the scheme as a whole: all staff involved in the scheme are required to report on their activity and these reports are integrated by the scheme manager who receives advice from the scheme board.

AN EARLY EVALUATION OF THE SCHEME

The following review of information gathered through questionnaires and interviews with students, lecturers and managers is offered to give a feel for the scheme in action.

The overall response is very favourable. All concerned agreed that the range of units available is comprehensive and enables the development of an individual programme that is relevant and applicable to the student's own practice. Flexibility is valued, although students and teachers comment that it can be overwhelming and even demotivating unless adequate information and guidance are available.

Unit timetabling is complex: a balance must be achieved between offering too few units to provide choice and offering so many that student numbers are too small to make them viable. Their order and timing is based on guestimates of student requirements and, given the diversity of their previous experience, this is a complex task and requires a sophisticated administrative infrastructure that at present is still in development. Students report that there are spaces in their programmes because no relevant unit is running and other periods when the units overlap. However, on balance students and lecturers and employers prefer to retain the flexibility that would be lost if a more easily administered system was introduced.

Managers have proved to be supportive to students and they can envisage a potential change in practice as a result of the scheme. However, as one manager points out, the individual may change and wish to change her\his practice, but major change is a result of many interrelated factors and may take time to come about. The degree of manager involvement in programme planning varies and reflects the individual's style. In one partnership the manager also gives feedback on the student's written work, and textbooks, as well as ideas, are exchanged. Managers and students prefer the newly introduced late afternoon and evening teaching sessions: though tired after work, students felt better able to combine work and study. One manager commented that she no longer sent students on 'traditional' courses because: a) they left no room for choice and were expensive, whereas this scheme recognized previous learning, related learning to work and was more cost-efficient; b) learning experiences in the scheme were deemed to be consistent with adult education philosophies and had increased general confidence – students appreciated the opportunity to undertake critical evaluation of their practice and were helped to understand empowerment within the profession.

Lecturers report that they have been able to 'exercise and develop their creative skills' and have experienced an increase in satisfaction within the teaching role. They comment on the high level of student motivation and the wealth of experience that leads to spontaneous participation in tutorials and seminars. They find the 'new' type of student stimulating and challenging. They recognize and have responded to a need to provide a study skills unit to support students making the transition to higher education study.

The issue of studentship and membership of a wider student group is also raised by the lecturers. The diverse nature of individual programmes means that students are unlikely to meet as a cohort and the sense of belonging to a student body is reduced.

Some units are designed to recruit students from other professions and voluntary and community groups, but the specialist and vocational nature of the programme may limit the broadening of horizons experienced by other students in higher education. This may also perpetuate the conflict felt by the student who is also a worker.

From what we have learnt we are now in an ideal position to move into the next phase, that is, to tap into a much wider market. The scheme has been shown to be flexible enough for overseas students to consider planning trips to England to undertake relevant units and complete their pathway. The whole concept has been well received by students and local purchasers of education. This is demonstrated by an increasing number of applicants and a continued commitment confirmed through the contracting process.

REFERENCES

Benner, P. (1984) *From Novice to Expert*, Addison Wesley, California.

Bloor, M. and Butterworth, C. (1990) Realising human potential. *Aspects of Education Technology*, **24**.

Butterworth, C. (1992) More than one bite at the APEL – contrasting models of accrediting prior learning. *Journal of Further and Higher Education*, **16**(3).

CNAA (Council for National Academic Awards) (1987) Credit Accumulation and Transfer Regulations, CNAA, London.

Davies, C. (1990) *The Collapse of the Conventional Career – The Future of Work and its Relevance for Post-registration Education in Nursing, Midwifery and Health Visiting*, English National Board for Nursing, Midwifery and Health Visiting, London.

Dearden, G. (1991) *The Credit Rating of In-company Courses, HMSO, London.*

ENB (English National Board for Nursing, Midwifery and Health Visiting) (1991) *Framework for Continuing Professional Education for Nurses, Midwives and Health Visitors: Guide to Implementation*, ENB, London.

Eraut, M. (1992) Developing a professional knowledge base: a process perspective on professional training and effectiveness, in *Learning to Effect – Annual SRHE Conference*, (ed. R.A. Barnett).

Foreman-Peck L. (1993) Enterprise education. *Vocational Aspects of Education*, **45**(2), 99–111.

Further Education Staff College (1989) *A Guide to Work Based Learning Terms*, Further Education Staff College, Blagdon, Avon.

Gibbs, G. (1988). *Learning by Doing – A Guide to Teaching and Learning Methods*, Further Education Unit, London.

Gorringe, R. (1989). *Accreditation of Prior Learning Achievements: Developments in Britain and Lessons from the USA*, Further Education Staff College, Blagdon, Avon.

Jarvis, P. (1983) *Professional Education*, Croom Helm, Beckenham, Kent.

Jessup, G. (1991) *Outcomes: NVQs and the Emerging Model of Education and Training*. The Falmer Press, London.

Kolb, D. and Fry D. (1985) Towards an applied theory of experiential learning, in *Theories of Group Processes*, (ed. C. Cooper), John Wiley & Sons, Chichester.

Kremer-Hayon, L. (1990) Reflection and professional knowledge, in *Insight into Teachers' Thinking and Practice*, (eds C. Day, M. Pope and P. Denicolo), The Falmer Press, London.

Land, R. (1991) *Rationale for a PGCE*, Thames Polytechnic Validation Office, London.

Otter, S. (1992) *Learning Outcomes in Higher Education*, Unit for the Development of Adult Continuing Education, London.

NCVQ (National Council for Vocational Qualifications) (1991). *Guide to National Vocational Qualifications*, NCVQ, London.

Schon, D. (1983) *The Reflective Practitioner – How Professionals Think in Action*, Basic Books, London.

SEEC (South East England Consortium for Credit Accumulation and Transfer) (1990) Report of National Conference on CATS in Practice held May 1990. SEEC, London.

UKCC (1990) *Report of the Post Registration Education and Practice Project*, United Kingdom Central Council for Nursing, Midwifery and Health Visiting, London.

<table>
<tr><td>4</td><td># Case study: Physiotherapy Access to Continuing Education</td></tr>
</table>

4

Case study: Physiotherapy Access to Continuing Education

Alan Walker and John Humphreys

Editors' introduction

This case study illustrates a rapid national transition in which a non-linear open curriculum structure is applied to meet local clinical needs. In this context the orthodox concept of course coherence is replaced by student-centred coherence worked through a mechanism of 'statements of intent'.

THE HISTORICAL CONTEXT OF PACE

Physiotherapy is a practical profession where the term 'hands-on' has a literal meaning. It follows that physiotherapy education has always been firmly rooted in practice. PACE, or Physiotherapy Access to Continuing Education, is a pioneering scheme for post-registration study and professional development that subscribes fully to the principle of practice-centred education. Yet its introduction in 1990 by the Chartered Society of Physiotherapy and subsequent development in collaboration with the University of Greenwich have been aimed as much to remedy the historical weaknesses of practice-based education in the post-registration arena as to build on its strengths.

The profession of physiotherapy is 100 years old, being founded in 1894 as the Society of Trained Masseuses. It was granted a royal charter in 1920 and adopted its present title, the Chartered Society of Physiotherapy, in 1942. State registration for physiotherapists followed in 1960. Physiotherapy is defined in the Society's 1991 curriculum of study as 'a health care profession which emphasizes the use of physical approaches in the prevention and treatment of disease and disability' (CSP, 1991a). Chartered physiotherapists are employed in a wide range of settings, from NHS acute and community units to private practice, sports clinics, independent hospitals and occupational health.

The Chartered Society of Physiotherapy is the recognized professional, educational and independent trade union body for approximately 24 000 chartered physiotherapists within the UK. It has five main groups of functions:

1. setting and maintaining educational, ethical and professional standards;
2. supporting members and their professional activities;
3. performing a trade union function on behalf of employed members;
4. acting as the voice of the profession;
5. providing services to members.

The society's function in supporting educational opportunities and standards is paramount. In pre-registration study, the society works in collaboration with the state registration body, the Council for Professions Supplementary to Medicine, in recognizing and validating courses leading to initial qualification as a physiotherapist. In post-registration study, the society has since 1990 developed the PACE scheme as its principal means of encouraging and accrediting continuing education opportunities for its members.

The rationale of PACE must be understood within the context of professional and educational developments during the past 20 years. As with other health care professions, the training of physiotherapists was based entirely in hospitals until recent times. In 1970 a review committee of the Chartered Society of Physiotherapy recommended that physiotherapy education should include the opportunity for graduate qualification (CSP, 1970). It was not until six years later, however, that the first undergraduate degree in physiotherapy was established in the University of Ulster. Significantly, the main impetus for degree-based education occurred in Northern Ireland and Scotland, where the transfer of physiotherapy schools from the NHS to the higher education sector had largely taken place by the early 1980s. In England and Wales, a governmental embargo prevented the development of physiotherapy degrees and as late as 1988 only two had been established. The majority of physiotherapists qualified instead via a national examinations system operated by the Chartered Society of Physiotherapy with the society's own award, the Graduate Diploma in Physiotherapy. After the embargo was removed, a period of explosive development in physiotherapy education followed. Between 1989 and 1992 24 physiotherapy degrees were established in the UK, and the profession became all-graduate by entry in September 1992.

The context of health and educational provision

An important corollary of the above development was the widespread transfer of physiotherapy education to the higher education sector. For the first time this placed the study of physiotherapy in a multi-disciplinary and research-based context. But even now, the transfer was less complete in England and Wales than in Northern Ireland and Scotland. In 1993, a total of 13 schools of physiotherapy still remained in the NHS sector, despite possessing accreditation links with higher education institutions for the purpose of degree validation. Crucially, the government's *Working for Patients* NHS review of 1989 yoked the planning and funding of health care education to the Department of Health rather than the Department of Education. *Working Paper 10: Education and Training* identified Regional Health Authorities as responsible for assessing future workforce demands in health care and commissioning the education and training required (Department of Health, 1989). Although higher education was becoming increasingly responsible for the delivery of courses in health care, this responsibility was tempered by an overall 'employer-led' concept of education.

Working Paper 10 must also be seen in the context of the 'internal market' created in both the health and educational sectors at the end of the 1980s. The *Working for Patients* review established a framework of 'purchasers' and 'providers' within the health service, including self-governing trust hospitals and budget-holding general practitioners. At the same time, the abolition of the 'binary line' between universities and polytechnics, and the consequent liberalization of course approval procedures, meant that higher education institutions became more entrepreneurial in their approach to course provision.

The growth of a market economy in health and education had a significant effect on schools of physiotherapy, which were now obliged to tender for educational provision at the behest of regional health authorities. As a result of this process, eight schools were decommissioned between 1989 and 1993 and four new schools established, all of them in higher education. At a later stage, this market economy would also have an important bearing on the development of PACE and continuing education generally.

Professional priorities in education

The historical development of pre-registration study in physiotherapy during the 1970s and 1980s did not in general stimulate the growth of continuing education within the profession. The former location of training within the NHS meant that schools of physiotherapy were isolated from the wider framework of higher education and had no corporate or financial incentive to expand their existing provision. The schools therefore identified themselves wholly with initial qualification and took little or no part in planning and operating post-registration courses. Moreover, the battle to achieve degree level education, and subsequently, to survive the implementation of Working Paper 10, preoccupied many schools of physiotherapy to the exclusion of post-registration or postgraduate concerns.

This heavy emphasis on pre-registration study was echoed in the Chartered Society of Physiotherapy, where before 1982 there was comparatively little discussion of continuing education issues. In that year, the society's council approved the establishment of a Post-Registration Education Committee for this purpose, but significantly, it was constituted on an entirely separate basis from the main Education Committee. This led to a continuing division between pre- and post-registration perspectives within the society's educational policy-making.

The demand for continuing education

Nevertheless, a considerable demand for continuing education had built up within the profession. This reflected significant changes within physiotherapy which came to fruition during the 1980s, despite the apparent lack of educational advancement at that time. The first of these was the growth of autonomy within the profession. Physiotherapists assumed responsibility for the diagnosis of patients, rather than simply carrying out treatments under the direction of medical practitioners. The second change related to the development of specialisms and specialities within the profession. Some of these specialisms related to clinical treatments, for instance those in manipulation and neurology, while others, such as paediatrics, were related to a specific client group. In 1987 the society's council formally recognized these specialties by creating clinical interest groups (CIGs). By 1993 these had grown to a total of 20, and were becoming an increasingly important focus of participation by members of the Society.

The climate was therefore favourable for continuing education initiatives which emphasized the autonomy of the physiotherapist as both learner and practitioner, and exploited the new specialist areas of study. With the exception of the Open University and a few other institutions, however, the needs of physiotherapists remained largely unmet in higher education during the 1980s. In the absence of a higher education response, the responsibility for setting up long, practice-based post-registration courses therefore fell on clinicians themselves.

The characteristics of practice-based continuing education

These courses, mainly developed from the mid-1980s onwards, were characterized by their location in hospitals rather than schools of physiotherapy or higher education institutions. Although physiotherapy teachers were sometimes involved in the courses on an individual basis, the bulk of teaching and assessment was carried out by clinicians. This model of course development, conducted apart from higher education, had many strengths. Not least of these was the ability to establish clinical courses quickly according to perceived need, together with the evident authority of the course tutors in their particular subject specialties. In the longer term, however, the model contained critical weaknesses, which may be summarized as follows.

1. The lack of educational involvement led to the teaching and assessment methods of some courses being didactic in approach, allowing insufficient opportunity for reflection on the part of the students.
2. The lack of educational infrastructure meant that practice-based courses were dependent on those clinicians who were prepared to devote personal time and energy to their design and teaching.
3. The lack of any external validation or quality control meant that no academic recognition could be given to those physiotherapists who successfully completed clinical courses.

The role and policy of the CSP

The role of the society in continuing education from the mid-1980s, culminating in the PACE proposals, became steadily more proactive. In May 1984, the Post-Registration Education Committee published a policy statement committing the society to a vigorous role in defining and initiating a structured post-registration education system to take physiotherapy into the 21st century (CSP, 1984). The first fruits of this new role was the publication of a discussion paper, *The Development of a System of Post-Registration Education for Chartered Physiotherapists*, which was circulated to members along with a questionnaire in order to elicit views on the future development of post-registration education (CSP, 1985a).

The responses, published by the society in 1986, revealed that physiotherapists required an expansion in the number of clinically based courses validated by the CSP, more academic courses in higher education and, above all, a nationally structured system of post-registration education, ensuring that education and training opportunities were widely available to encourage staff mobility and satisfy individual and employer needs (CSP, 1986).

In line with the society's proactive policy, the growth of practice-based courses led in 1984 to the professional validation of post-registration courses according to national criteria. By 1985, 10 such courses had been successfully validated, and guidelines for post-registration validation were published by the society (CSP, 1985b). A small number of courses also obtained academic status from associated higher education institutions during the 1980s.

The post-registration education master plan

The responses and aspirations of physiotherapists were addressed more fully in January 1988 by the publication of a post-registration education master plan. The aim of the plan was to make continuing education more accessible to physiotherapists, and it mapped out all the ways in which physiotherapists could continue their education (Titchen, 1988). Members of the society welcomed the plan, in particular its recommendation for a mixture of clinical and academic routes to postgraduate education. It was also felt, however, that the plan was too complex and should be simplified.

By this time, the Education and Post-Registration Education Committees had combined, and post-registration study received a higher profile within the society's educational work as a whole. In July 1989, the Education Committee set up a working party to devise a practical scheme for putting the master plan into operation. The title of the working party's report, when presented and subsequently published in 1990, was *Physiotherapy Access to Continuing Education* (Walker, 1990). The framework of continuing education which the report proposed has since adopted the acronym of its title: PACE.

The PACE report acknowledged both the strengths and weaknesses of continuing education in physiotherapy and, while it was built on the philosophy of the 1985 discussion paper and the 1988 master plan, it went beyond the work of its predecessors in setting out radical approaches to implementation. The overall priority switched from the formulation of a comprehensive educational model to the creation of a robust system capable of introduction within a rapid timescale. The tempo of development in continuing education quickened accordingly during the next two years.

THE PRINCIPLES OF PACE

PACE started from the recognition that education was a continuing and lifelong process that could take many forms, not all of them traditional. The rate of social and technological change was such that an initial period of professional education could only provide the disciplinary foundations of knowledge and skills, on which further education and experience must be built if they were to remain current and valid. Education itself might serve as an agent of this change, as with the growth of undergraduate degree programmes, while organizational reforms already referred to, such as the establishment of an internal market within the NHS, provided further impetus for professional development.

These external changes interacted with developments occurring within the profession to form a matrix of continuing education needs. The growth of autonomous practitioners would be a prerequisite for the transfer of NHS services from hospital to community settings, for example, while undergraduate education would create a market for higher study which further extended the model of the autonomous and reflective practitioner.

The context of change placed great responsibility, therefore, on the existence and encouragement of continuing education, and on the individual physiotherapist for undertaking further study. The disadvantages inherent in the model of practice-based education outlined above, however, meant that the scarcity of courses and their lack of recognition acted as a deterrent to further study. The need for a flexible and versatile structure within continuing education was therefore paramount.

The society also sought to establish and clarify a desirable profile and balance in continuing education. This would be particularly valuable in a clinical profession where, as already indicated, many specialist areas of practice were emerging. It was important to legitimize specialist study in the eyes of employees and the profession alike. Equally, in a time of change and greater individual responsibility for physiotherapists, it was vital to promote more general areas of study which transcended professional boundaries. Above all, post-registration study needed to stress the continuum of education and the value of experiential learning.

Contemporary developments in education

In its PACE proposals, the society was therefore concerned both to map out the territory of continuing education in physiotherapy and to provide a flexible system by which permanent and widespread recognition could be given to studies undertaken. Contemporary developments in education gave further credence to the society's emphasis. The introduction of credit accumulation and transfer schemes (CATS) and national vocational qualifications (NVQs) in the mid-1980s laid great emphasis both on the value of all forms of continuing education, whether academic, practical or experiential, and on the need to recognize these various endeavours by the most flexible means.

In the case of CATS, the society already possessed a vehicle for transforming its plans into reality. The PACE system was built explicitly on a credit accumulation structure. This had twin advantages: first, a physiotherapist would be able to build up credit on a gradual basis for studies undertaken; and second, these studies could reflect a learning profile unique to the individual, combining different types of continuing education. It therefore became an operating principle of PACE that any component course must receive a credit rating as part of its recognition.

The Diploma in Advanced Physiotherapy Studies

At the heart of the original PACE proposals was a new award to be issued by the society: the Diploma in Advanced Physiotherapy Studies. This was an open award, not attached to any particular course, but gained by credit accumulation through a negotiated learning programme. To obtain the award, a physiotherapist needed accumulate at least 120 credit points from a programme that exhibited a coherent balance between practice-based courses, the general studies referred to above and assessed experiential learning. It was expected that the 120 points would be gained over a maximum period of five years, though this period would be flexible, allowing for career breaks or a change of employment. It would break down into the component parts shown in Figure 4.1.

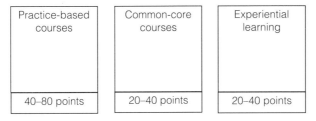

Credit 120 points (minimum of 40 at level 3)

Figure 4.1 Structure of Diploma in Advanced Physiotherapy Studies.

The practice-based courses included the clinically based courses previously validated by the society, together with similar courses operated by other bodies. Examples of these were courses designed for physiotherapists working in manipulation, respiratory care and occupational health. In order to establish credit ratings for these courses, the society introduced a new process of course accreditation, which replaced the validation system hitherto operated. A new Post-Registration Accreditation Panel was designated to fulfil this function. By adopting a CATS system, it was possible to recognize and accredit courses of varying length, depth and type.

The category of 'common-core' courses encompassed a wide range of relevant general and non-clinical subjects. Most of these were offered by higher education institutions as part of CATS Level 3 or Level M programmes, and included areas such as management, research, teaching and counselling. It was not intended to accredit these courses directly, since this would duplicate the accreditation process already undertaken by higher education institutions. Rather it was proposed to accept the institutions' own credit ratings within the PACE framework, provided the course was relevant to the continuing education needs of physiotherapists.

Experiential learning naturally had a wide potential remit, and at the time of the original PACE proposals in 1990, the society had yet to develop an overall policy for its recognition. This task was devolved to a newly formed Experiential Learning Working Party, which did not report until 1991.

It will be noted that no requirements were originally enforced in respect of credit point levels for the Diploma in Advanced Physiotherapy Studies. At its outset, the PACE system very much represented a lateral, practice-based route of study. It was not proposed, for instance, that M Level study should be included in the scheme. The society aimed to encourage the development of physiotherapy-related courses at postgraduate and Master's level, however, and the PACE scheme was intended to forge closer collaboration between clinical course teams and higher education institutions.

THE OBJECTIVES OF PACE

In launching the PACE system, the Society wished above all to develop continuing education on a flexible basis. PACE was intended to meet the needs of all physiotherapists, whether in the public, private or voluntary sector; whether newly qualified, returning to practice or changing career direction; whether developing specialist clinical skills, working with a client group, or qualifying as a teacher. The individualized learning programme would provide an exact profile of a physiotherapist's background, experience and qualifications. The society believed that, by providing a clear outline of required study and a greater reward for those who successfully completed it, it would be possible to convince more employers of the significance and value that post-registration study represented, while physiotherapists themselves would be more inclined to pursue it.

In summary, therefore, the original objectives of PACE were as follows:

1. to encourage physiotherapists to take responsibility for their own learning and continue their professional education throughout their careers;
2. to provide a structure of post-registration and continuing education that could meet the educational needs of physiotherapists at any stage of their careers;
3. to provide permanent and widespread recognition for studies undertaken, in particular by creating links between post-registration study and the higher education sector;
4. to emphasize practice-based learning that was responsive to service needs;
5. to encourage flexible and accessible modes of learning.

Problems of credit rating and academic currency

Almost from the start, however, there were seen to be problems in the proposals for credit rating within the PACE scheme. The society had launched the Diploma in Advanced Physiotherapy Studies as a practice-based award carrying professional recognition. At the same time, it wished to promote access to higher education programmes by means of advanced standing for PACE accredited courses. This would be of particular interest to those physiotherapists who qualified by means of the society's own Graduate Diploma in Physiotherapy. The latter was credit-rated in the CATS system at only 240 points at a maximum of Level 2, as opposed to 360 points at a maximum of Level 3 for an honours degree.

It was accepted that no chartered physiotherapist would have any academic need for Level 1 or 2 credits, as they would have already gained the maximum total of 240 points in these levels by virtue of their initial qualification. By contrast, Level 3 courses would confer general credit which could be claimed towards a degree award, as well as the society's own diploma. For these reasons, the Post-Registration Accreditation Panel was prepared to award credit points at Levels 1 and 2, even though it had no academic authority to do so. In the case of practice-based courses at Level 3, however, the panel advised that these should be validated and credit-rated by higher education institutions.

This arrangement was soon revealed to be cumbersome and illogical. Many practice-based courses were submitted to the panel requesting accreditation at a mixture of Levels 1, 2 and 3, while others were unwilling to seek accreditation from higher education institutions. This was often because the accreditation fees of the institutions were prohibitive, or because the mobile nature of some courses, capable of delivery in hospitals up and down the country, militated against local links with any one institution.

In addition, the work undertaken by the Experiential Learning Working Party highlighted specific problems of academic currency. It was decided that all experiential learning undertaken within the PACE system must be accredited at a minimum of Level 3, since such learning represented the summation of professional development and could not reasonably be rated below the level of final year Honours – at which many physiotherapists were beginning to qualify. This decision raised the immediate question of how Level 3 experiential learning could be accorded wider academic currency, since the society envisaged this component as an integral part of its own diploma.

These problems were compounded by the fact that some diplomate physiotherapists misinterpreted the diploma as conferring an academic status it did not have. It became clear that the Diploma in Advanced Physiotherapy Studies needed to be more firmly related to the hierarchy of academic awards in the credit accumulation and transfer system. By the end of 1990, the basic framework of PACE had been established, but the lack of academic authority for the credit points issued by the society was identified as a barrier to further development.

The search for academic partnership

At first it was envisaged that the society might seek accredited status from the Council for National Academic Awards for the award of credit points within PACE. It was already apparent by this time, however, that the future of the CNAA was uncertain, and accreditation arrangements would have to be made directly with higher education institutions in future. In addition, accredited status from the CNAA would not directly assist the society in developing its expertise in accreditation, as the society would still be undertaking this activity on its own. It was clear that a closer partnership with higher education was required.

At this point the society was approached by the University of Greenwich (then Thames Polytechnic), expressing interest in PACE. As part of the PACE launch, the society had circulated publicity literature to a range of higher education institutions with the hope of involving them in some aspect of the proposed scheme. Among the latter was the University of Greenwich, with whom several meetings were now arranged.

Discussions with the University of Greenwich

Discussions with the university were centred on the School of Post Compulsory Education and Training (PCET), one of three schools within the University's Faculty of Education. The school was interested in the PACE scheme as a whole, which mirrored closely its own work in credit accumulation and the accreditation of prior learning, particularly in the health studies and teacher education fields. At first, discussions were concerned with the possibility of recognizing the society's Diploma in Advanced Physiotherapy Studies with a specific credit value towards one or more postgraduate awards offered by the university.

The feasibility of creating a Master's degree in physiotherapy was questioned by the society's Education Committee, however, given that the majority of the profession had limited knowledge of research methodology or actual research experience. It was also felt that only a small proportion of the society's membership would wish to engage in postgraduate study, and that the Diploma in Advanced Physiotherapy Studies would constitute the post-registration award of principal interest for the present time (CSP, 1991b).

These views are significant in retrospect, given that the first Master's degrees in clinical physiotherapy were starting to be validated, and that the profession's interest in Master's study as a whole exploded during the early 1990s. They do, however, underline the rapid transition in educational development and philosophy that occurred in physiotherapy during this time, and which PACE would in many respects crystallize.

Collaboration and accreditation

The society agreed instead to give priority to the creation of a joint mechanism with the University of Greenwich whereby components of the PACE scheme could be credit-rated simultaneously on a joint academic and professional basis. The advantages of this arrangement were as follows.

1. The relationship between the society's Diploma in Advanced Physiotherapy Studies and the hierarchy of credit accumulation and transfer was clarified. All credit points within the PACE scheme were academically valid as CATS general credit.

2. The society would be working in collaboration with an institution which had substantial experience and expertise in the areas of credit accumulation and transfer and the accreditation of prior learning. This was a benefit not available through accreditation from the CNAA, and proved helpful to the society in tackling the theoretical and practical problems of credit rating.
3. It was possible to give general credit at Level 3 to experiential learning undertaken within the PACE scheme.

Despite these advantages, the wisdom of creating a formal accreditation link with a single higher education institution was questioned by some, especially as the University of Greenwich did not contain a school of physiotherapy.

It was pointed out, however, that the university was being approached for its educational expertise in accreditation, rather than its knowledge of physiotherapy, which would be provided by the society itself. While the logic of the society's partnership with the University of Greenwich was eventually accepted, and work towards a formal Memorandum of Co-operation began, misgivings at its seemingly exclusive nature persisted among other higher education institutions. The need to encourage these institutions to become involved in PACE ultimately led to the creation of the PACE Consortium of Higher Education Institutions in 1992.

The third stated advantage of the new partnership, relating to the granting of credit to experiential learning, was extremely important given that the society's Experiential Learning Working Party had now completed its report (CSP, 1991c).

Experiential learning

The working party started from the premise that, in a clinical profession, all learning must ultimately be judged by its practical value. Experiential learning, or learning by doing, described any professional experience which led to learning or development in some form. The Working Party set down the following criteria for the recognition of experiential learning within PACE.

1. Learning should be clearly differentiated from experience. Knowledge, understanding and skills were assessed for credit, not for what had been done or experienced.
2. Knowledge, understanding and skills should be current. While the experience may have occurred at any time, it was necessary to demonstrate the current application of any learning being claimed.
3. Learning should demonstrate general transferability outside the specific situation in which it was acquired.

4. Learning must be at a level appropriate to the credit accumulation and transfer scheme.

The working party did not favour experiential learning taxonomies such as Benner's progression 'from novice to expert' (Benner, 1984), or the definition of professional competencies as a means of measuring experiential learning. The use of these systems would have severely restricted the flexibility of the PACE system, which was designed to facilitate rather than prescribe. In particular, it would prove impossible to apply taxonomies to the wide range of prior experience undergone by physiotherapists. Neither did the working party favour pre-set learning contracts within the individualized PACE scheme. Rather, it recommended the production of a 'statement of intent' by students in respect of their identified programmes of experiential learning.

The statement of intent

The statement of intent was designed to give an outline of the prospective package of study towards the Diploma in Advanced Physiotherapy Studies, and the learning objectives for which accreditation would subsequently be claimed. It would also relate the proposed experiential learning to the wider learning programme through PACE, including details of practice-based and common-core programmes which the physiotherapist intended to undertake.

In line with the original principles of PACE, the experiential learning component was regarded as work-based; hence the support of employers would be explored and confirmed as far as possible when preparing the statement of intent. It was believed that experiential learning could complement existing in-service development, for example, by formalizing the process of senior I physiotherapists' supervision of junior staff. While many in-service programmes were unsuitable for accreditation as free-standing programmes, they could be incorporated into experiential learning programmes and serve as a stimulus to more detailed independent study.

The Professional Development Diary

This early work by the society in the area of experiential learning had an important spin-off for the profession. The society became aware of the work of a group of physiotherapists at the Royal Hallamshire Hospital, Sheffield, who had begun work on a professional diary in which the progress of experiential learning could be recorded. The society decided to endorse this development, and put the physiotherapists in touch with its consultant in experiential learning, who was based at Sheffield Hallam University. The resulting diary was widely piloted at 24 sites throughout the UK, including NHS hospital and community services in inner city and rural areas, self-governing trusts, industry, independent hospitals and private practice. In all, 175 physiotherapists took part in the pilot process.

The Experiential Learning Working Party remained in existence until 1992 to oversee the pilot period. The diary was amended and improved following feedback from the pilot sites. As a result, the CSP Professional Development Diary was launched at the Royal Hallamshire Hospital in September 1992 and subsequently marketed by the Society (Watson and McManus, 1992). The working party recommended that while the diary had made a valuable contribution to the PACE scheme, in particular by providing a means to record experiential learning and shape the raw material for a subsequent portfolio and accreditation claim, it should be used in a wider context than PACE alone.

The diary was seen as a valuable professional tool which facilitated the setting of personal and professional objectives, and could play a key role in the development of physiotherapists as reflective practitioners. The Professional Development Diary was henceforth promoted as a document with career-long relevance, and in 1993 it was further agreed that the diary should be issued to all student members of the society at the commencement of their undergraduate study. This byproduct of PACE thus found its own role in the forward development of the profession.

The joint accreditation arrangement

Work progressed rapidly towards an accreditation arrangement between the Chartered Society of Physiotherapy and the University of Greenwich, and a document was prepared for validation by the two partners in July 1991 (CSP and University of Greenwich, 1991b). The rationale for the arrangement was presented in terms of the need to provide academic currency, as well as professional recognition, for the PACE scheme. This was an extension of the society's proactive role in meeting the needs of its members.

These needs were evident in two ways. First, the rapid transition to all-graduate pre-registration education, then in its spate, was bound to increase the interest in higher study by qualified physiotherapists. Second, the demand for academic recognition was particularly acute among holders of the Graduate Diploma in Physiotherapy.

This demand had hitherto been met by the study of 'top-up' or 'end-on' health studies degrees, which provided the 120 points at Level 3 required for the award of a degree with honours. These degrees were offered on a multi-disciplinary basis by a number of higher education institutions in the UK. While many physiotherapists took advantage of this route, they involved a great deal of employer support that could not necessarily be given, and once completed, might represent a practitioner's only opportunity for extended further study. Many physiotherapists desired academic credit to be given for other forms of continuing education, including practice-based courses and experiential learning in the workplace.

The demand for academic credit within PACE was therefore forecast to centre on both Levels 3 and M, in terms of Graduate Diploma holders wishing to upgrade towards a degree, or physiotherapy graduates and diplomates wishing to claim advanced standing towards one of several postgraduate awards.

As already explained, many practice-based courses operated outside the higher education sector were unable to develop formal links with higher education institutions. The accreditation arrangement therefore proposed that the credit rating of these courses should be organized on a joint basis between the society and the University of Greenwich. The general credit conferred through the link with the university would provide academic recognition for practice-based courses outside the higher education system, via the credit accumulation network in the UK. It was also intended that the partnership between the society and the university should be extended to the accreditation of individual experiential learning within the PACE scheme. This would overcome the difficulties envisaged by the Experiential Learning Working Party in granting credit points with academic currency for experiential learning at Levels 3 and M.

The objectives of the accreditation arrangement

In summary, the objectives of the accreditation arrangement were as follows:

1. to ensure that educational activities operated outside the higher education system but included within the PACE scheme, whether formal courses of study or experiential learning, were given both academic and professional currency by means of joint credit-rating between the society and the university according to the national credit accumulation and transfer network as originally formulated by the Council for National Academic Awards;
2. to encourage physiotherapists to undertake courses of higher and postgraduate study, in particular by affording academic credit for clinical, general and experiential study successfully completed within the PACE scheme;
3. to promote a national network for the development and recognition of the PACE scheme, in particular by securing the involvement and participation of other higher education institutions, professional bodies and training agencies.

The third paragraph largely reflected the concerns of the society that the links with Greenwich should not be seen as exclusive. In reality, the accreditation arrangement had little to do with this work, which eventually became the remit of the PACE Consortium of Higher Education Institutions in 1992. The involvement of other higher education institutions was welcomed, however, both as providers of 'common-core' material and as accreditors of practice-based courses. Because the majority of common-core courses originated in higher education institutions, this area of provision was largely excluded from the accreditation arrangement. At a later stage, though, accreditation for such courses was sought by higher education institutions without access to CATS mechanisms, and by some clinically based course teams.

The management of the accreditation arrangement

The accreditation arrangement between the Chartered Society of Physiotherapy and the University of Greenwich was managed under the terms of a Memorandum of Co-operation agreed between the two partners (CSP and University of Greenwich, 1991a). The memorandum set out the parameters for collaboration between the society and the university, including the objectives of the agreement, the role of each partner, administrative and financial agreements, and mechanisms for disputes, annual review, and termination.

The centrepiece of the memorandum was the Joint Post-Registration Education Panel. This panel comprised representatives of both the society and the university, and reported simultaneously to the society's Education Committee and the Academic Standards Committee of the university. The society was accustomed to dealing with committees of dual parentage, and the panel was modelled after the Joint Validation and Recognition Panel in undergraduate education, where the society worked alongside representatives of the Council for Professions Supplementary to Medicine.

There were some significant differences, however, between the two panels. These were designed to offset the perceived problems in linking with a single higher education institution. First, the total membership of the panel had an inbuilt majority of Society representatives, ensuring that the Society could not be outvoted on any matter by the university.

Second, the management structure for PACE accreditation was so arranged as to ensure that the partnership with Greenwich did not preclude the involvement of other higher education institutions in PACE. Post-registration courses in physiotherapy could be accredited directly by higher education institutions with a representative of the society present, so enabling their inclusion within the PACE scheme. There were thus two routes to PACE accreditation, with the partnership with Greenwich being intended, as already stated, to accredit courses without higher education links, together with individual experiential learning.

An organizational implication of the above was that several of the society's continuing post-registration functions, such as monitoring courses operated by higher education institutions and receiving reports of their validation activity, would lie outside the scope of the Memorandum of Co-operation. It was therefore decided to maintain the society's own Post-Registration Education Panel alongside the Joint Panel operated with the University of Greenwich. The society membership of both panels, including the chairmanship, was common. A diagram showing the separate lines of responsibility for the two panels, and the twin routes to PACE accreditation, is shown in Figure 4.2.

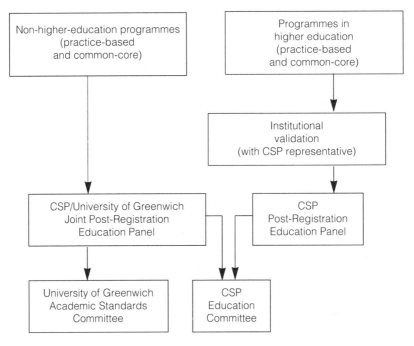

Figure 4.2 Management structure for PACE accreditation.

The Memorandum of Co-operation required the Joint Post-Registration Education Panel to submit a review of its activity to the society's Education Committee and the university's Academic Standards Committee at the end of each academic year. This was seen as an important means of monitoring the success of the partnership, as well as summarizing the year's activity. Overall, the memorandum made it clear that the administration and development of the PACE scheme, including the conferment of the Diploma in Advanced Physiotherapy Studies, remained wholly with the Chartered Society of Physiotherapy.

Criteria for accreditation

Nevertheless, the influence of Greenwich was already accelerating the forward development of PACE. Even before the validation of the arrangement in July 1991, joint work on accreditation had commenced. Perhaps the most significant

event was the workshop sessions held between society and university representatives in June 1991, which identified criteria for the award of credit levels
within the PACE scheme. For the first time, the postgraduate M Level was regarded as part of the overall framework.

Learning at the different levels of the PACE structure could now be separately characterized. As the criteria included Levels 1 to 3, they were based on
the philosophy of the undergraduate curriculum of study published by the
society in January 1991. The different Levels were included in the July 1991 accreditation document (CSP and University of Greenwich, 1991b), and were
defined as follows.

Level 1 encompassed the 'building blocks' of knowledge and competence that
contributed to becoming a professional physiotherapist. It was concerned with
those basic aspects of science and professional studies set out in the curriculum
of study.

Level 2 learning was focused on the patient and the relationship between the
physiotherapist and the patient. It was concerned with the integration of science
and professional studies into this professional context, and the application of
these to patient care.

Level 3 was concerned with the higher-order professional abilities that charac-
terize the graduate physiotherapist. It was focused on the physiotherapist as an
autonomous practitioner and encompassed the development of research skills. It
was also concerned with the ability to make professional assessments and diag-
noses, solve problems and justify professional action.

Level M learning contained two elements. It comprised both learning in greater
depth than the curriculum of study, in the areas of clinical knowledge, management, research or education. It also involved the ability to advance the physiotherapy profession in one of these four areas through making use of analysis,
critical thinking and problem-solving skills.

Another influence of the university's involvement was felt in the preparation
of regulations for the Diploma in Advanced Physiotherapy Studies, and the joint
accreditation of courses and experiential learning. For the first time this codified
the process of diploma registration. The society also fixed the requirements for
credit point levels within the diploma. From the total of 120 points, a minimum
of 40 was required at Level 3 and a maximum of 80 at Levels 1 and 2. Claims
for experiential learning had to be made at a minimum of Level 3.

THE WORK OF THE JOINT POST-REGISTRATION EDUCATION PANEL

Following the successful validation of the accreditation arrangement, the Joint
Post-Registration Education Panel was formally constituted in September 1991

and met on a quarterly basis henceforth. During its first year of operation, the panel successfully accredited a total of 23 continuing education programmes. Fifteen of these were courses already recognized within the society's former validation system, while eight, encouragingly, were wholly new. The accredited courses spanned a wide range of practice areas, including acupuncture, obstetrics and gynaecology, and care of the elderly. The panel was, however, unable to recommend the accreditation of several courses and modules. Advice and guidance were provided to the course teams concerned on how their courses and documentation should be developed to permit accreditation.

Two of the courses considered by the panel were given accreditation at Level M. It was felt that these courses differed substantially from other submissions which had been considered, in particular in their requirement for students to review their existing knowledge in the light of new research presented within the course. The Level M courses also encouraged a strongly evaluative and critical approach to learning, and one of the courses had an expectation that students' research findings would be suitable for publication.

Consideration was given by the panel to ways of assisting course teams in preparing submissions. Written guidelines on requirements for accreditation were revised and circulated to course teams, who were encouraged to seek the involvement of both educationalist and physiotherapist advisers in the development of their courses. Annual study days for course tutors were already a regular feature of the society's work, and these now began to focus on issues of quality assurance and linkage with higher education.

Scrutineers and the course monitoring process

Course monitoring procedures were perceived as an integral and ongoing part of the accreditation process. In view of difficulties experienced with the standard of monitoring reports, it was decided to introduce a system of assigning two scrutineers from the Joint Panel to each course in receipt of accreditation. The primary function of scrutineers was to monitor the running of a particular course through the course team's and external assessor's reports submitted on each student intake. Particular attention was paid to whether a course's aims and objectives had been met. If a report failed to provide an adequate level of evaluation, the scrutineer contacted the course team directly. The scrutineers also reported their findings to the panel, thus informing the panel's feedback to course teams.

Crucially, if the monitoring reports brought into question the validity of the original credit-rating, the course team would be invited to re-submit the course for accreditation. The 'scrutineer' system proved successful and influential, with a similar process being introduced by the society's and CPSM's Joint Validation and Recognition Panel for undergraduate physiotherapy courses.

Problems of general and specific credit

Just as the original PACE proposals were rapidly overtaken by the need to gain academic authority for the society's accreditation activity, so the launch of the accreditation arrangement with the University of Greenwich was upstaged by pressure from the society's membership regarding the award structure within the PACE framework.

The existing arrangement between the society and the university was for the provision of general credit, i.e. the academic value attached to an item of learning by a single higher education institution. The possibility of obtaining specific credit for PACE, whereby learning obtained within the PACE scheme would count towards one or more academic awards offered by the University of Greenwich, was first mooted at the joint validation event in July 1991. The issue gained greater urgency as a result of two events: the society's 1991 Annual Representatives' Conference and the opening of registration for the Diploma in Advanced Physiotherapy Studies.

The following motion was approved by the Society's Annual Representatives' Conference in September 1991: 'The CSP should continue with the principle of Physiotherapy Access to Continuing Education (PACE), but suspend the Diploma in Advanced Physiotherapy Studies until something more academically rewarding can be arranged' (CSP, 1991d). Although the motion was proposed without knowledge of the accreditation arrangement with the University of Greenwich, the basic sentiment received widespread support even when the scope and function of the arrangement were outlined. This could be largely explained by sensitivity among the membership regarding degree and diploma qualifications. As already stated, the aspiration of many physiotherapists was to gain a degree in addition to their existing graduate diploma. In this context, the original concept of PACE as a lateral, practice-based route of study which led to a diploma award was not regarded as attractive in academic or professional terms.

The society's response

While the society's council declined to withdraw the diploma, it was clear that PACE needed to be aligned to specific academic awards. This message was reinforced by the disappointing level of recruitment to the Diploma in Advanced Physiotherapy Studies. Responses from enquirers revealed that the validity of the diploma was being questioned, both in terms of its relation to academic awards and its potential for enhancing career prospects. Many physiotherapists expressed a preference for embarking on academic awards such as 'top-up' or Master's degrees, rather than undertaking study towards a professional qualification.

The society now had to respond to newly expressed needs which had emerged from the introduction of PACE itself. Fortunately, the accreditation arrangement with Greenwich was flexible enough to create a system capable of meeting these needs. Further integration between the PACE scheme and higher education structures would now be required.

Discussions began between the society and the university regarding the establishment of two academic routes of study within PACE. These were identified as a 'top-up' honours degree worth 120 points at Level 3 and a postgraduate diploma worth 70 points at Level M. Work on the postgraduate diploma soon ceased, however, as it was considered too ambitious to introduce two academic awards simultaneously.

THE BSc(HONS) PHYSIOTHERAPY STUDIES

The BSc(Hons) Physiotherapy Studies, as the 'top-up' degree became known, was designed as a radical, self-directed programme of professional learning, offered end-on to society membership and leading by means of credit accumulation to the award of an honours degree. The rationale for the degree was twofold: to empower individual physiotherapists in their professional learning and development, and to meet the academic aspirations of non-graduate physiotherapists.

The honours degree was centred on the model of the physiotherapist as an autonomous and reflective practitioner, as it was believed that such practitioners would be increasingly required in physiotherapy practice (CSP and University of Greenwich, 1992). The programme of learning therefore involved a primary relationship between physiotherapists and their professional practice. The curriculum model of the honours degree, involving self-directed learning, individual research and credit accumulation, was designed above all to extend the practice of physiotherapists in a reflective and investigative manner.

The aims of the BSc(Hons) Physiotherapy Studies were as follows:

1. to foster the development of practising physiotherapists as autonomous and effective professionals;
2. to enable physiotherapists to plan, negotiate and implement a programme of self-directed learning that was responsive to their own needs and those of the service;
3. to develop the ability of physiotherapists to evaluate and reflect on their own professional practice by means of balanced and coherent learning programmes;
4. to extend the powers of physiotherapists critically to investigate aspects of professional practice by means of a synoptic research project.

The use of an open curriculum

The BSc(Hons) Physiotherapy Studies differed from conventional 'end-on' degrees in that it was based on an open curriculum. It did not comprise a formal

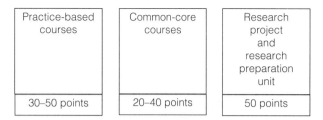

Figure 4.3 Structure of BSc(Hons) Physiotherapy Studies.

academic curriculum to be studied in linear fashion, but rather a learning programme obtained and accredited within the PACE framework, allied to mandatory research units. Prior learning of various kinds could also be claimed for accreditation in this package. As with the degree's predecessor, the Diploma in Advanced Physiotherapy Studies, the specific learning programme would be unique to the individual physiotherapist. The honours degree, however, took the philosophy of self-directed and practice-centred learning further than it had ever gone before within the context of physiotherapy studies, or even in health care education as a whole.

Because the points total of a 'top-up' honours degree was the same as that for the Diploma in Advanced Physiotherapy Studies (120 points), it was possible to transfer the internal PACE structure of practice-based courses, common-core courses and experiential learning to the new degree proposal. The degree differed from the diploma, however, in so far as the category of experiential learning was now expressed in terms of research activity. The internal structure of the honours degree is shown in Figure 4.3.

Practice-based and common-core components

The practice-based and common-core course categories remained much as they had been within the Diploma in Advanced Physiotherapy Studies. There was now a wider range of these courses available within PACE: 22 practice-based courses and 141 common-core programmes were recognized within the structure. Some adjustment was made in the points ranges required for these categories, however, in order to incorporate a mandatory research project.

It was also a requirement that these categories of courses should be accredited at Level 3, comprise a minimum of 30 hours learning and contain formal assessment of students' learning gained through their undertaking the course. Providing the statement of intent formed a balanced and coherent learning programme at the appropriate level, the credit value of practice-based and common-core programmes was treated as advanced standing on a specific basis, and therefore granted in full towards the honours degree.

The research project

The research project took the place of experiential learning as the third component within the revised PACE structure developed for the BSc(Hons) Physiotherapy Studies. The degree remained practice-based in nature, however, and it was expected that physiotherapists would draw heavily on their work and professional experience in furnishing the raw material for the project. The university and the society also developed a preparatory unit for use in connection with the project.

The research preparation unit was principally designed for those physiotherapists who qualified via the former national examinations system and had thus received little exposure to formal research methods in their pre-registration education. Students undertaking the project needed to have an understanding of research methodology and the ability to assess the appropriateness of individual methodologies as applied to particular subjects of study. Although intended for a specific clientele of students, it was suggested at the validation of the degree that all students should be required to undertake the research development unit.

As the research project and the associated preparation unit were the only components of the honours degree to be supervised and assessed by the University of Greenwich itself, the overall credit rating was fixed at 50 points, rather than operating within a range. In this way the project could be supervised and assessed on a consistent basis. While this meant that only 50 points were directly assessed from the total of 120 in the programme of learning (and 360 in the honours degree as a whole), the integrating function of the project served to ensure that all aspects of professional learning within the degree were expressed through this component, and thus informed the assessment of the honours degree. The final outcome of the research project was a dissertation of between 10 000 and 12 000 words.

Accreditation of prior experiential learning

In addition to the major components of the honours degree, physiotherapists were able to claim accreditation for prior experiential learning (APEL), whether gained informally in the professional setting, or through undertaking courses not accredited in the PACE scheme. Accreditation of prior experiential learning was designed to complement the overall philosophy of the course, whereby physiotherapists took responsibility for the direction and balance of their learning programme.

Prior experiential learning was presented by means of a portfolio, which indicated how the learning was comparable with that achieved through attendance on a recognized course. The credit rating of a portfolio was evaluated by means of the definitions of levels previously established by the society and the university. APEL could be accrued to a maximum of 40 credit points in lieu of either practice-based or common-core units, but the research project remained mandatory and could not be thus exempted.

Problems of educational coherence

The structure and philosophy of PACE, with its self-directed learning programme, adapted well to the nature and demands of an honours degree. Specific problems had to be resolved, however, in the potential lack of coherence inherent in a programme of learning drawn from widely varying sources. There was a natural tension between the principles of an honours degree and those of credit accumulation. The former emphasized the precise academic grading of directly taught material, while the latter stressed the successful completion of study at a broadly defined level, often by means of prior learning obtained elsewhere. These tensions were not easy to resolve, but several strategies were adopted to reconcile the problems arising from the flexibility of the open curriculum model.

It was first recognized that the key to coherence in a self-directed programme of study lay in the transfer of responsibility for the learning process to the student. Those who undertook this degree would be mature professionals able to establish and meet their own learning needs. Students on the BSc(Hons) Physiotherapy Studies were therefore required to complete a statement of intent in respect of their proposed learning programme. This statement of intent, modelled after that used in the Diploma in Advanced Physiotherapy Studies, was designed to elicit the internal coherence of the learning process and programme. Students were expected to demonstrate that the individual learning components shared a common theme and direction, and reflected the balance of study inherent in the honours degree structure. The statement of intent included the following elements:

1. an outline of the prospective learning programme, demonstrating its overall credit level, direction and balance;
2. the projected timescale for its completion;
3. the elements for which accreditation would subsequently be claimed, i.e. the practice-based and common-core courses the physiotherapist intended to undertake;
4. any prior learning which the member wished to claim for accreditation, and the taught course elements which would be exempted as a result;
5. the intended nature of the research project and its relationship to the taught courses and/or prior learning.

The second strategy was to draw on the existing strengths of the accreditation arrangement between the society and the university. Because the Joint Post-Registration Education Panel acted both as a quality control agency and overall supervisor of the honours degree, it was possible to ensure that the practice-based and research components were truly of Level 3 standard, and of relevance to the continuing education needs of physiotherapists. The potential problem of the honours degree becoming a 'patchwork' of varying quality and depth was therefore minimized. In this way, the new phase of collaboration between the society and the university can be seen as dependent on their previous joint activity.

The use of distance learning techniques

The organization of the BSc(Hons) Physiotherapy Studies was planned jointly by the society and the university on a distance learning basis. The principal new resource involved the appointment of a Programme Director to assume day-to-day management of the honours degree. The Programme Director was respons-ible for recommending the approval of learning programmes, the supervision and assessment of research projects, and the assessment of APEL claims. All these functions made the maximum use of distance learning techniques. The re-search project and preparation unit could be undertaken by any physiotherapist within the UK without the need for face-to-face tuition. Counselling and assess-ment for APEL was carried out on the same basis.

Support from the society was given by means of centralized registry and ad-ministrative services, together with the Information Resource Centre, which had been opened for the benefit of members in 1991. This comprised a substantial collection of professional journals, databases and bibliographical services. Students on the BSc(Hons) Physiotherapy Studies programme were encouraged to make use of the centre's resources, which could again be accessed on a dis-tance learning basis by post, phone or fax.

The use of distance learning techniques allowed a wide geographic and occu-pational range of students on the course. It should be noted that educational iso-lation was not only caused by distance from higher education institutions, but also by the nature of a professional's occupational and personal circumstances. These factors were particularly acute in a profession which contained an over-whelming proportion of women and a significant number of private practition-ers. Distance learning techniques were therefore valuable to students whose time and commitment were at a premium. The first students enrolled on the course were based in widely distant parts of the country, and the BSc(Hons) Physiotherapy Studies could be regarded as a truly national scheme, albeit linked to a single higher education institution.

The role of the existing partnership

The management of the degree was based firmly on the existing Memorandum of Co-operation between the society and the university, which was updated ac-cordingly. Overall responsibility for supervision and coordination of the degree was conferred on the Joint Post-Registration Education Panel, whose role was expanded to act as a scheme board and scheme board of examiners. The panel had responsibility for overseeing the application of the degree's regulations and their administration, ensuring that a close relationship was maintained between the component parts of the scheme, and that the philosophy of the PACE scheme and the academic standards of the University of Greenwich were maintained through the delivery of the honours degree.

The panel retained the same membership as before, except that the Programme Director became an additional University of Greenwich representative, while a student representative was also present on the panel when acting in the role of a scheme board. In addition, the chairman of the Scheme Board of Examiners was provided by the University of Greenwich. The constitution of the Joint Panel ensured that effective collaboration occurred between the society and the university regarding the operation of the degree.

Parallel developments in higher education

Before 1992, only limited interest had been expressed in the PACE scheme by higher education institutions other than the University of Greenwich. Several institutions submitted individual modules or entire programmes of study for recognition as 'common-core' material within PACE, but despite extensive publicity, no other institution had put itself forward as a direct provider of either the Diploma in Advanced Physiotherapy Studies or the BSc(Hons) Physiotherapy Studies.

This may have been partly due to the perceived exclusive arrangement between the society and Greenwich but, nevertheless, new trends were beginning to emerge in respect of postgraduate and post-registration study in the higher education sector. The first was the establishment of Master's degrees in physiotherapy. These were often developed by individual schools of physiotherapy in association with their parent higher education institutions, notably King's College and University College, London, the University of East London, Coventry University and the University of Manchester. Many of these programmes were wholly physiotherapy-centred, sometimes in a particular specialty, while others were more generically based in health studies, with specific physiotherapy routes identified within them.

The second development was the establishment of more general post-registration programmes by schools of physiotherapy. These included practical programmes such as courses designed to prepare clinical supervisors of undergraduate students for their role and work. Many schools of physiotherapy were also beginning to form links with practice-based course teams outside the higher education system. This had two advantages: course teams were able to benefit from the educational expertise of higher education institutions, while the educational infrastructure of institutions was often able to provide a more secure basis for the operation of such courses. This was important, since the increasing emphasis on contracts and costing within the NHS was threatening the survival of courses operated on the basis of goodwill and individual commitment. The clientele for these courses was also being squeezed by the curtailment of study leave and financial support by employers for continuing education.

The expansion of post-registration study by schools of physiotherapy may also be seen as a response to the internal market created in the health and education arenas. Given that schools and their parent higher education institutions were now dependent on regional health authority contracts, post-registration and post-graduate courses provided a valuable diversification of educational output. In a similar way, higher education institutions not involved in undergraduate physiotherapy studies identified a possible expansion of their market in postgraduate studies for physiotherapists. By 1993 the market for continuing education was much more open and competitive than it had been during the previous decade.

THE PACE CONSORTIUM OF HIGHER EDUCATION INSTITUTIONS

Given the stated intention of PACE to develop into the postgraduate sphere and encourage links between individual course providers and higher education institutions, it was clear that the PACE scheme needed to encourage the participation and contribution of these institutions on a more systematic basis. In March 1992 the society convened a conference on 'Credit Arrangements with Higher Education Institutions'. The purpose of the conference was to establish support in higher education institutions to develop both PACE and postgraduate schemes in physiotherapy generally. At the end of the conference, the society suggested that the creation of a consortium of institutions involved in the delivery of PACE would be valuable, in particular by facilitating the creation of a credit transfer system. This suggestion was endorsed by many of the institutions present, and later by the Education Committee of the society, which welcomed approaches being made to other interested higher education institutions to become more involved in the delivery of PACE.

The PACE Consortium of Higher Education Institutions met for the first time in April 1992, and by 1993 comprised 22 institutions. Because PACE was a custom-built credit system for physiotherapy studies, the criteria for membership of the consortium stated that each higher education institution should normally have a CATS policy that enabled it to offer academic awards on the basis of credit accumulation and transfer, together with access to physiotherapy expertise in order to ensure the professional credibility of PACE study routes. Where such a route was operated by a member institution, a nominated course leader for the PACE programme was also required.

It should be noted that membership of the consortium required 'access to physiotherapy expertise' rather than formal linkage to a recognized school of physiotherapy. Some of the strongest interest in the PACE scheme was expressed by higher education institutions with no prior involvement in pre-registration physiotherapy education, but which operated post-registration and postgraduate programmes of study for several health care professions on a multi-disciplinary basis. The University of Greenwich, a founder member of the consortium, itself fell into this category. A total of eight institutions within the consortium contained no school of physiotherapy, and some of these began to appoint physiotherapists expressly in order to expand their overall commitment. This could be seen as a tangible benefit of the PACE initiative.

The role and functions of the consortium

The PACE Consortium defined its terms of reference as follows:

1. to develop the PACE scheme through participation by higher education institutions;
2. to establish a common understanding on issues of accreditation policy;
3. to recommend principles for the recognition of modules/courses accredited in the PACE scheme as specific credit;
4. to encourage good practice on the principles and methodology for the accreditation of prior experiential learning (APEL);
5. to provide a networking function to encourage good practice through the sharing of knowledge.

Many of the discussions held by the consortium were designed mainly to share information or consider common problems, but the first major initiative of the consortium involved a decision that members would accept the credit-ratings of all courses recognized within PACE as specific credit, subject to the individual physiotherapist's learning programme forming a coherent educational package. This decision resolved one of the persistent problems of credit accumulation and transfer schemes, where higher education institutions only gave partial recognition to the general credit from learning obtained elsewhere, so that the specific credit actually given was often substantially less.

A second major development within the consortium was the establishment of other BSc(Hons) Physiotherapy Studies programmes in member institutions. These programmes were modelled after the scheme developed by the Society and the University of Greenwich, but unlike the Greenwich scheme, were not free-standing. Instead they comprised specific routes through wider 'top-up' degree schemes, and were endorsed directly by the Society through its Post-Registration Education Panel. By 1993 two of these programmes had been introduced, at Leeds Metropolitan University and Anglia Polytechnic University. Other member institutions began to plan similar schemes.

An Assessment of PACE

By 1993 the BSc(Hons) Physiotherapy Studies operated by the society and the University of Greenwich was firmly established. The accreditation arrangement between the two partners also continued, and after its second year of operation, the Joint Panel had directly accredited 32 programmes. In addition, the society had recognized a total of 288 modules and courses operated by higher education institutions. The cohesion of the panel developed considerably over its first two years, and much mutual benefit was derived from the respective expertise that each partner brought to the accreditation process.

In retrospect it is possible to define four distinct phases in the development of PACE: the original 1990 proposals relating to the Diploma in Advanced Physiotherapy Studies; the accreditation agreement between the society and the University of Greenwich in 1991; the development of the BSc(Hons) Physiotherapy Studies in 1992; and the subsequent creation of the PACE Consortium of Higher Education Institutions. Each of these phases has been dependent on the work undertaken in preceding periods. While these developments are still too recent to offer a final analysis, it is clear that PACE has been extremely successful in developing accreditation and credit transfer systems, both via the agreement with Greenwich and in the wider arena of the consortium.

This has had beneficial effects for the standards and availability of continuing education. Accreditation offers a precise tool for standard-setting, in that course proposals are considered against specific criteria for levels of credit, rather than the more vague and general standards of normal course validation. It also highlights the importance of educational processes within course provision, as opposed to the traditional concern of professional validation with course content and structure.

It is clear that the partnership between the society and Greenwich has acted as a 'magnet' in attracting other higher education institutions to become involved in PACE. This expansion of continuing education opportunities was at the heart of the original rationale for the PACE scheme, but it was not until the joint accreditation process had commenced on a large scale, and the plans for the honours degree had been announced that higher education took serious note of PACE and the marketing potential it represented. PACE has now become a useful 'brand name' for higher education, employers and physiotherapists themselves.

In other ways, also, higher education was able to benefit from the pioneering accreditation activity undertaken by the society and the university. The PACE consortium, with its ambitious scheme for the mutual recognition of specific credit, would not have been possible without the initial work of the Joint Post-Registration Education Panel. As the society began to shape its strategy for the development of the postgraduate M Level within PACE, a new emphasis has been placed on creating open learning opportunities of all kinds in continuing education, and increasing the mutual recognition of these learning opportunities by higher education institutions. The role of the consortium will clearly be vital and instrumental in pursuing these aims.

In terms of its own definition, PACE has proved itself successful. As a case study, it demonstrates how a professional body can meet the needs of its members as created by external factors, and subsequently address further needs which the initiative itself had generated. The main innovation of PACE has been its extreme flexibility, which has permitted the forward development of the scheme when circumstances demanded. It has also created a facilitating framework for post-registration study, with an emphasis on the processes of education in all its forms.

PACE has undoubtedly increased access to continuing education by physiotherapists, through extending the recognized boundaries of study, developing an open learning curriculum, and creating firm links between the needs of practice and the opportunities of higher education. PACE will continue to offer new possibilities in embracing the postgraduate developments of the future.

ACKNOWLEDGEMENTS

The authors would like to acknowledge the assistance of Diane Kinsella, Sally Gosling and Thelma Harvey of the Chartered Society of Physiotherapy in preparing this chapter.

REFERENCES

Benner, P. (1984) *From Novice to Expert*, Addison Wesley, California.

Chartered Society of Physiotherapy (1970) Report of the CSP Review Committee. *Physiotherapy*, **56**(6), 264–270.

Chartered Society of Physiotherapy (1984) Post-registration education – policy statement. *Physiotherapy*, **70**(5), 183.

Chartered Society of Physiotherapy (1985a) The development of a system of post-registration education for chartered physiotherapists – a discussion paper. *Physiotherapy*, **71**(8), 360–362.

Chartered Society of Physiotherapy (1985b) *Guidelines for the Validation of Post-Registration Courses*, CSP, London.

Chartered Society of Physiotherapy (1986) The development of a system of post-registration education for chartered physiotherapists – a response from the membership. *Physiotherapy*, **72**(7), 373–374.

Chartered Society of Physiotherapy (1991a) *Curriculum of Study*, CSP, London.

Chartered Society of Physiotherapy (1991b) Minutes of the Education Committee, 16 Jan 1991, para. 33–39, pp. 6–8.

Chartered Society of Physiotherapy (1991c) Report of the Experiential Learning Working Party, Education Committee, 17 Apr 1991.

Chartered Society of Physiotherapy (1991d) Motions for debate, Annual Representatives Conference 1991. *Physiotherapy*, **77**(7), 468.

Chartered Society of Physiotherapy and the University of Greenwich (1991a) Memorandum of Co-operation between the Chartered Society of Physiotherapy and Thames Polytechnic, July 1991.

Chartered Society of Physiotherapy and the University of Greenwich (1991b) Proposed Accreditation Arrangement between the Chartered Society of Physiotherapy and the University of Greenwich, July 1991.

Chartered Society of Physiotherapy and the University of Greenwich (1992) Proposed BSc(Honours) Physiotherapy Studies, July 1992, vol. 1, p. 5ff.

Department of Health (1989) *Working Paper 10: Education and Training*, HMSO, London.

Titchen, A. (1988) The development of a post-registration education master plan. *Physiotherapy*, **74**(1), 10–12.

Walker A (1990) Physiotherapy access to continuing education – credits for a new diploma. *Physiotherapy*, **76**(9), 537–538.

Watson, A. and McManus, M. (1992) *Professional Development Diary*, Chartered Society of Physiotherapy, London.

Case study: marketing professional development in education

5

Ray Land and John Humphreys

Editors' introduction

This third case study describes a full marketing approach to the development of initial training (for teachers). The study illustrates how the principles of client-centred development, programme flexibility and team responsiveness are not restricted to continuing post-experience professional development. Of the three curriculum development case studies described, this one corresponds most completely to the development model described in Chapter 9.

The post-compulsory education sector includes all education beyond the school leaving age, encompassing health care education, higher, further and adult education. The training of teachers for this sector has occurred in two main modes, pre-service and in-service. Pre-service teacher training is aimed at suitably qualified professional and commercial personnel who wish to teach in the post-compulsory sector on completion of a Certificate in Education or Postgraduate Certificate in Education course. In-service teacher training, on the other hand, is aimed at individuals who are already employed as teachers within the sector, but who do not possess a teaching qualification.

In September 1990 a decision was taken to go for an early review of a part-time in-service Certificate in Education (Further Education) course; although in-service, this constituted initial training. The course at that time had been running for two years during which recruitment targets had been met and a favourable quality rating from HMI had been achieved. Although open to staff in any part of the post-compulsory sector, the major markets were in colleges of nursing and midwifery, further education colleges and adult education institutes. In addition to validation, the course had approval from the English National Board for Nursing, Midwifery and Health Visiting (ENB) which enabled health professionals to have their teaching qualification recorded by UKCC. Additionally ENB sponsored places were available.

Both the health and further education markets are characterized by primary and secondary client groups. In order to achieve recruitment both employee and employer must perceive the programme as addressing their needs. In addition to profound influence on the curriculum structure and design, this dual client feature also required carefully thought out promotional strategies. In the event, the new programmes sold vigorously on the basis of an 'overlapping interests' concept created by the advertising agency Austin Knight.

Additional major complexities included the fact that the course operated on a franchise in various colleges in London and south-east England, each of which had its own particular clients' needs, and therefore local focus, to attend to.

One of the many major decisions that had to be addressed by the development group concerned which features of the old course to retain. Being itself a recent development with ENB approval and a quality rating, the 'old' course had many merits. For example, it had benefited from a 'staged' structure consisting of four stages (I, II, Bridging and III) which corresponded to the nationally recognized ACSTT stages commonly applied in professional development for staff in adult education (ACSTT, 1978). However these stages and the spiral curriculum principle underpinning them put limits on flexibility and responsiveness. In the event, market research provided the answer.

Despite some progress in recent years, the understanding and application of principles of marketing is still very patchy in post-compulsory education and training (PCET). Senior managers in PCET can still be heard on occasion to equate marketing with advertising or wider promotion strategies. In such circumstances many institutions and/or departments are likely to continue to neglect markets and clients to the point of organizational decline. In the absence of understanding of marketing, some organizations will have no hope of addressing the real implications of a marketing approach with regard to the role of staff in curriculum development. In the context of the present development, the speed and appropriateness of change was underpinned by a market-led, client-centred ethos established over the preceding years. The flaws of product-centredness and production-centredness which were characteristic of traditional 'academic' establishments were not apparent in the development team. Furthermore a climate of innovation and calculated risk tolerance made the process stimulating, as well as productive. This climate had already over the previous four years led to the development of a sophisticated and successful CAT scheme based on a credit accumulation framework designed collaboratively within the Faculty of Education. This framework, designed specifically to enable high-quality professional development for education practitioners, was a significant aspect of the context of development. In the event, the introduction of initial (Certificate level) work into the framework constituted the final component of its development. Broad details of the framework have been reported elsewhere (Hall, 1991; Butterworth, 1992; Butterworth and Bloor, 1989).

MARKET RESEARCH

Three sources of information provided our market intelligence in the subsequent development of the new programme. These might be categorized as follows.

Primary sources

Our initial consultation was with the client group of the existing certificate course. The clientele comprised a range of interested parties, as discussed below.

The concerns and recommendations of existing students were elicited from annual course reports of previous years and through regular course monitoring procedures, including representation on centre course committees. The existing cohort of students, as part of their study of curriculum design issues, took part in a major review of the course. The curriculum design component of the existing course was brought forward to allow a self-selected student curriculum design group to make specific contributions to the development process of the new programme as their chosen option and work in tandem with the actual development team. This student group submitted proposals at various stages through to the validation event which they attended as observers.

The changing needs and priorities of client organizations were clarified through questionnaires, a conference convened early in the course design process for vice-principals, heads of department and staff development officers, and a series of nationally advertised open forums held at monthly intervals. Presentations were given by senior management at individual institutions, particularly those such as Havering College of Further and Higher Education which operated as the centre of a consortium.

Secondary sources

A series of consultations with other providing institutions and national agencies helped shape our understanding of the wider national perspective. The national conference *The Search for Continuity in Further Education Teacher Training*, held at Huddersfield Polytechnic on 25 February 1991 brought together a wide spectrum of teacher educators with officials from the CNAA, the CGLI and HM Inspectorate. Our presentation at the event provided a useful opportunity to subject our developing curriculum at that point to the criticism and advice of peers.

An earlier conference at the CNAA in late December 1989 had alerted the existing course providers to the possibility of credit accumulation at Level 1 for certificate courses and the notion of a ladder of awards. During the course design process in 1990-91 consultations were held with the CNAA to discuss the definitions of levels of professional awards, to consider the possibility of credit transfer to BA (Education and Training) awards, to suggest a range of available titles to accompany awards and to assess the degree of flexibility that might be attained within CNAA regulations concerning hours of study and patterns of attendance.

In late December 1990 a conference was organized jointly by the English National Board for Nursing and Midwifery (ENB) and the CNAA to consider the developing needs of tutors within the health professions. Members of our course design team who attended this conference were alerted to the strong preference of ENB for recognition of the postgraduate status of many of their tutors. The ENB, as a national agency governing the practice of a sizeable proportion of our clientele, was consulted in February 1991 to test reaction to the more radical features of our emerging course design and to ensure that these would be compatible with requirements for United Kingdom Central Council (UKCC) recognition of our health professional students. A conjoint validation was agreed for the following May.

Tertiary sources

Early in 1991 the visit of HMI Christine Frost to our BA (Education and Training) programme as part of a nationwide review of credit accumulation provided an opportunity to refine further the notion of professional, as opposed to academic, levels of study, leading to a clearer understanding of what was to be a crucial distinction in our eventual programme between study levels 1 and 2 .

The information gleaned from these various sources also helped us establish a clearer view of other significant issues. These included the funding realities within which the course and its clientele would have to operate, the demand from the market for increased flexibility, what would constitute appropriate unit coverage, the likely effects of the relinquishing of the old 'Haycock' Stages and the political climate prevailing within the PCET sector.

Conclusions

It became apparent from these consultations that the provision of training within the sector had been affected by three principal factors:

1. an atmosphere of declining resource and continuing financial stringency;
2. the increasingly effective in-house provision of INSET by client institutions;
3. the sustained pace of curriculum and organizational change within the sector.

These factors led to an awareness by the course design team of the growing demand for an increased flexibility in provision which could facilitate a range of course design features whilst ensuring the maintenance of standards. For example, students needed to be able to build up to awards through a variety of attendance patterns and modes of study. New course elements needed to be designed and incorporated swiftly. Acknowledgement needed to be given to the professional development being undertaken within client institutions and to the value of collaboration between such institutions and higher education providers.

The market research also precipitated a number of decisions. It was agreed that the avoidance of prescribed content, which was a feature of the original course, would be retained. The notion of institutional focus, according to which all coursework was designed to have practical application to the course participant's employment experience would similarly be retained, but as part of an endeavour to link course activity with real-time professional developmental needs rather than any hypothetical envisaging of these needs. Self-managed learning would be further developed. Block attendance would be abandoned. Statements of competence would be used to a limited degree. (These were restricted to Level 1 – see below – but with the advent of national TDLB standards were later developed into a portfolio with full competence specifications requiring range statements and performance evidence.) The notion of stages would be dropped but applicants possessing Stage II of the City and Guilds 7307 or ACSET would be eligible to receive up to 60 credit points of the 120 point total of the new scheme. The distinction between two-year part-time day modes and four-year extended modes of study would be abandoned and their respective weekly teaching requirements of 10 hours and four hours be replaced by an overall supervised teaching experience (STE) requirement of 200 hours by completion of the course. This would be akin to the notion of 'flying hours' required for the pilot's licence and would require line manager verification.

CURRICULUM DEVELOPMENT AND DESIGN

The process of development

Five factors seem to have been significant in determining the modus operandi of the development team.

1. **External regulations:** There was a tension during the course development between the perceived needs of both providers and clients and the formal constraints presented by external regulatory authorities of bodies such as the CNAA and the ENB. An example of this was the non-recognition by the ENB of the status of the City and Guilds 7307 which severely curtailed the credit accumulation facility available to many health professional tutors entering the programme.

2. **University of Greenwich credit accumulation framework (CAF) regulations:** A similar debate was held internally in order to extend the existing CAF regulations to accommodate a CertEd/PGCE programme within the scheme. Whereas internal persuasion and consultation generally led to amended regulations, such as a new definition of levels to include work levels 1 and 2, other proposals had to be dropped. The original intention, for example, to keep STE out of formal units was ceded to the CAF requirement that any assessed activity must be capable of carrying credit.

3. **Five-year commitment rule:** The composition of the development team was intended to include members from all networked colleges offering our courses. A rule requiring a commitment from colleges to remain within the Thames Polytechnic INSET Network for the first five years of the new programme's operation led to three colleges having to withdraw from the development process.

4. **Structure of development teams:** The development teams comprised a core team of six members representing the three institutions operating the new programme. This core was supported by three satellite teams, one in each institution. The notion of core and satellite teams had been put into practice a year earlier in the development of a new pre-service certificate course. The course director of the in-service programme had been brought into the core team of this earlier development for staff development purposes and was later able to adapt this structure.

5. **Working process:** Proposals emanating from the core team were reported back to satellite teams in the institutions who discussed them with colleagues and students and in turn reported back to the core team. Papers often criss-crossed between the institutions between meetings with objections, amendments or new proposals. Tasks were allocated among members of the course team to be completed with the help of their satellite teams and brought back to the core for further consideration.

The eventual success of the development process and the relatively smooth operation of the teams seems to have been attributable in great part to the way in which the limited size of the core group assisted decision-making. The pattern of task allocation led also to a sense of responsibility and ownership and the use of satellite teams not only aided the dissemination of innovative ideas but fostered involvement and a feeling of representation. On the few occasions when the development process reached an impasse the contributions of colleagues, brought in on occasion to contribute their specialist experience or present a particular view, helped the team to reach a resolution. Communications were also undoubtedly assisted by the availability of fax machines for the swift transmission of documents – an important new tool in the process of curriculum development at a distance!

Product design

The certificate programme was designed as part of the credit accumulation and transfer scheme of the university (CATS). This enables course members to gain credit points by undertaking free-standing units of study. These units are offered at CATS Level 1 or Level 2, though it should be emphasized that these are levels of professional development and do not readily equate with the CNAA academic levels relating to the first years of an undergraduate degree. Experience has shown that course members with academic qualifications at Level M and beyond in their subject specialisms may be at the very start of their professional development as a teacher.

1. **Level 1:** This level encompasses the basic competences, skills, knowledge and understanding appropriate for an autonomous teacher/lecturer. It is concerned with learning that contributes to becoming such a person through a process of self-development involving action and reflection.
2. **Level 2** learning builds on Level 1 and involves study of these relationships in greater depth. This depth is achieved by requiring students to extend their knowledge through the use of a conceptual framework. An analysis of relevant existing theoretical and practical knowledge is required.

All units are predicated upon the understanding of a set of relationships fundamental to the teaching/learning process. The autonomous teacher/lecturer will need to understand the inter-relationships indicated in diagrammatic form in Figure 5.1.

Credit can be given for any learning that is at the appropriate level and furthers understanding of these relationships.

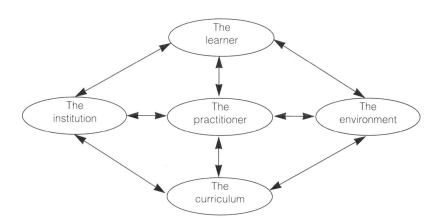

Figure 5.1 The network of relationships in the teaching/learning process.

Course rationale – competence and reflective practice

A continuing preoccupation of the course development team was the degree to which the notion of competence should inform the eventual curriculum and the model of the teacher that we were aiming to develop.

We were aware that effective performance in many occupations and professions requires the learning and use of necessary information, of standard procedures and routine skills. This kind of knowledge is an explicit feature of effective performance and lends itself to direct observation and assessment. It is commonly specified in terms of statements of competence and has been referred to as 'knowledge displayed in performance' (Eraut, 1990). It can be seen how certain aspects of teaching performance such as elements of lesson planning, demonstration of an appropriate repertoire of teaching/learning strategies, the preparation of learning resources and materials and effective operation of techniques of assessment might be so defined.

Members of the team knew from their own practice, however, that teachers in the post-compulsory sector are required to perform in a range of contexts, conditions and situations. In so doing they are confronted continually by the need to make judgements and decisions in relation to time, resources, learning need, interpersonal dealings, appropriateness of response, crisis and so forth. Priorities often conflict and must be resolved. Such decision-making, and the ability to adapt and modify performance as befits situations, draw on different kinds of knowledge which may not be directly apparent. Eraut distinguishes such knowledge and understanding as 'knowledge underpinning performance'. This kind of knowledge usually remains tacit in practice unless there is reason and opportunity for full discussion and justification of the decisions taken. Although it is harder to identify, such underpinning knowledge is clearly a significant component of effective professional practice and might well be deemed an essential quality in any definition of a fully competent teacher.

The current attractiveness of competence in relation to teacher development programmes has arisen partly from the legitimate societal demand for accountability. It focuses helpfully on the notion of teaching as skilful performance, requiring the use of practical intelligence. Nor is there any reasoned argument as to why skills defined in terms of competence should not be theory-imbued. For these reasons we felt that units offered at Level 1 of our scheme, addressing the needs of the less experienced teacher, were more helpfully offered in terms of statements of competence. Moreover members of our programme very often in their own practice find themselves obliged to operate competence-based schemes. Hence an understanding of such schemes gained experientially from a student perspective can only be beneficial.

Teaching in the post-compulsory sector, however, cannot in its wholeness be conceived as the sum of isolated effective teaching behaviours or skills. Competence, we felt, was a necessary condition of effective practice but not a sufficient one.

Given the current conceptual confusion in relation to competence we decided not to extend the concept to our Level 2 units but to work from the model of the reflective practitioner as described by Schon (1983) and others, with its emphasis on critical reflection and the application of theoretical intelligence and insight. This is not to imply that reflection is not required in the Level 1 units, nor that the two models are incompatible. Our level 2 units still seek to define clear learning outcomes, though with a greater degree of underpinning knowledge, and higher level professional competence, when eventually defined, may well resemble reflective practice. We saw the transition from one model to the other as a spectrum, a matter of degree. Level 1 is concerned more with notions of professional competence, (though still requiring reflection) and develops the 'competent practitioner'. Level 2 emphasizes critical theoretical intelligence, which is inseparable from the individual, and develops the 'reflective practitioner'.

Core/option

At each level students must complete a combination of four core and two option units. A wide range of options is available though it is also possible for course members to negotiate and design their own option units on a learning contract basis. This is done through the use of open units, and allows the student to tailor as much as a third of the programme to specific real-time concerns relating to her/his personal and professional development. A three-way partnership is encouraged in the planning of individual programmes which involves the practitioner, the employer and the university.

Awards

All units have a value of 10 credit points. A minimum of 60 credit points at Level 1 and 60 credit points at Level 2 are required for the award of the Certificate in Education. Graduates who gain 40 points at Level 1 and 80 points at Level 2 receive the Postgraduate Certificate in Education. An intermediate award, the Certificate in Teaching Competence, is available for those completing a programme of professional development at Level 1 and gaining 60 credit points. This may be represented diagrammatically in Table 5.1.

Table 5.1 Requirements of the different certificates in education awarded by the University of Greenwich

	Level 1	Level 2	Total
Certificate in Teaching Competence	60 points		60 points
Certificate in Education	60 points	60 points	120 points
Postgraduate Certification in Education	40 points	80 points	120 points

Each of these awards may carry one of the following titles depending on the locale of the student's teaching experience: Health Professions; Post Compulsory Education and Training; Further Education; Higher Education; Adult Education.

Through the principle of unit borrowing the programme permits students to take units from the BA (Education and Training) programme as option units. The CAF programme is also predicated on the idea of a credit ladder whereby Level 2 points gained beyond the minimum requirement may be transferred as credit towards a BA (Education and Training) degree.

Mode of study

Attendance patterns are flexible. Units may be achieved in any of four ways: 1) on a taught basis; 2) by distance learning; 3) through a negotiated contract; 4) by accreditation of prior experience and learning. Entry to the programme is possible at various points during the year.

APL/APEL

Credit can be given for appropriate learning through short-course attendance and previous relevant experience. Where prior learning has been gained through relatively recent attendance on award-bearing courses the accreditation is a comparatively straightforward process using a tariff of credit-ratings. Where accreditation is sought for the learning gained from a substantial seam of relevant professional experience students are encouraged to undertake an APEL option unit which will assist them to compile a professional development portfolio and submit a claim. Credit is given for attendance on this unit as on all others. This APEL unit has subsequently been developed through the use of open learning materials. (For a fuller discussion of the different approaches to APL and APEL in the Greenwich programme see Butterworth, 1992.) The maximum credit that can be given through APL or APEL is 50% (60 credit points).

Assessment

Assessment at Level 1 is undertaken through the meeting of competence requirements and the production of performance evidence. At Level 2 each unit in the programme is assessed by an assignment or task designed to further the personal and professional development of the student. All assignments are negotiated, have high professional relevance and a clear institutional focus. Students must also complete a reflective record for each unit based on the analysis of critical incidents and requiring them to integrate the theory acquired within a particular unit with their daily professional practice.

Validation

A conjoint validation was arranged with the ENB for 13 May 1991. The new programme was given approval with conditions, which subsequently were met. The unit validation facilities of the university's credit accumulation framework, however, allowed us to continue with the further development of the programme and within a month of the event we were able to submit further option units to extend the range of the programme.

Staff development

Despite the consultation with colleagues through the satellite teams the comparatively short time scale of the development process necessitated the immediate implementation of a tight schedule of staff development for all INSET staff who would be teaching on the programme the following September and for administrative staff having to deal with a growing stream of enquiries. Administrative personnel were now faced with the devising of a considerably more complex system of registration and record-keeping than before, though the experience of staff in establishing systems of credit accumulation for the BA (Education and Training) and MA degrees was of great value in this respect.

PROMOTING THE PROGRAMME

The marketing concept has implications for the approach to promotional and advertising campaigns. If market research is accurate and curriculum development consequently produces a desirable 'product' then subsequent promotional and advertising campaigns should disseminate, in an immediately accessible way, key features of the product which match market needs.

In the present context, the existence of primary and secondary clients – a complexity which strongly influenced the product design – also presented a challenge in advertising terms. Curriculum development work had produced flexible and relevant programmes which could meet the needs of individual lecturers while also addressing employers' organizational development, all within beneficial characteristics of price, pattern of attendance and sometimes place of delivery.

In the designing of a promotional strategy, the major issue was whether primary and secondary client groups should be targeted with separate promotional materials. After a briefing, the university's account director at Austin Knight Advertising came back with the view that the main selling feature of addressing both employer and employee needs could best be communicated by designing a single set of promotional materials in which the complementary positions of primary and secondary clients could be emphasized.

After further creative work at Austin Knight, a campaign based on the simple phrase 'overlapping interests' was proposed. The agency supported this advertising concept with a design for literature and posters based on an image of a face reminiscent of the figurative modern art of Picasso or Chagall. The face was a frontal view but with right and left sides separated by a curved profile running down the middle of the image. The overall effect was of two overlapping images which together formed a face that was simultaneously both single and double. This concept was further exploited in a leaflet design in which the two sides of the face were indeed overlapping front flaps of an opening leaflet. In this way, the concept of 'overlapping interests' was powerfully reinforced by both the image itself and the form of the leaflet.

In the event, the image of the face provoked much interest and various interpretations. In the first place the image was unconventional as an image for advertising higher education, which traditionally used simple text-only materials or conventional photography of students, computers or other facilities.

Additionally the two half faces (each half being similar in design but different in shade) have been interpreted as representing not only employer and employee (the original intention) but also student and teacher or black face and white face. These various dimensions to the image enhanced its ability to capture the potential client's interest, while maintaining a cultural and gender neutrality.

The day after successful validation, a co-ordinated campaign of mailshot, press advertising and personal contacting was implemented. At that time recruitment was low compared with previous years. Within weeks, recruitment had leapt, with additionally a number of serious enquiries from employers about local delivery and franchises.

UNRESOLVED CONCERNS

Inevitably the implementation of the new programme gave rise to unforeseen complications and difficulties. There were already certain lingering anxieties about the way in which certain issues would resolve themselves.

1. There could be a tendency for less scrupulous employers to exploit the flexibility of the scheme to gain an undue influence over the content of study and assignments of their staff attending the course.
2. The use of in-house mentors might be used or perceived as 'appraisal by the back door'; the all-important relationship of trust and confidentiality would be difficult to maintain if the mentor were also a line-manager.
3. R.S. Peters spoke of the 'paradox of freedom' when too much freedom can lead to too little. In a similar fashion our programme might give rise to a 'paradox of flexibility' through which too much flexibility in the scheme might allow local delivery centres to restrict the wide diversity of the scheme by closing off many of its options, thereby creating a closed curriculum less able to meet the market need.

4. Some students had already voiced their concern that the varied pattern of at-
    tendance might lead to employers withdrawing the provision of day-release.
5. Both delivery in local centres and study by distance learning might lead to
    students becoming comparatively isolated from their professional peer
    group. Contact with peers, of course, has often been shown to be a key
    source of innovative practice.
6. The development and introduction of distance learning materials was ini-
    tially beset by questions of timing and resourcing.
7. The operation of APEL, even through the medium of an approved option
    unit, might prove more costly in human resources than originally envisaged.
    There was also continuing discussion as to whether the process of reflection
    and analysis undertaken in the APEL process would elevate all learning in
    that unit to Level 2. Such a decision would have repercussions on other pro-
    grammes within the credit accumulation framework.
8. There remains an anomaly with the teaching requirements of our programme
    at Level 1 (100 hours) and that of the City and Guilds 7307 (30 hours). This
    does not help the process of establishing parity between the awards.
9. The demise and eventual disappearance of the CNAA has meant that there is
    no existing regulatory body to advise on establishment of appropriate levels
    for professional development in education and in a climate of competition
    and relative inexperience this might lead to inconsistency and unfairness to
    students in the transfer of credit between institutions.

CONCLUSION

The significant expansion (100+) of students at Level 2 in the first year of operation of the new scheme was felt to justify the intensive period of development
and to vindicate the features of the new design. In particular the removal of the
Bridging stage seemed to tap a source of recruitment which previously had been
impeded by the presence and timing of the Bridging stage. This tendency has
continued into the second year of operation of the programme.

The first year of the programme demonstrated the need for the development of
the original competence statements at Level 1 into a more fully-fledged form
that would incorporate range statements and descriptors of performance evidence. This was achieved by the beginning of the second year of operation as
was a Level 2 portfolio providing guidance on the writing of reflective records
and the writing of open units (learning contracts). The first year also saw the development and use of open learning materials for Level 2 core units. These have
now been systematically evaluated and revised for the second year of operation.
The APEL unit is now available through open learning materials and open materials for certain option units and Level 1 core units are being developed.

The demonstrated flexibility of the new scheme was eagerly exploited by
course members. Over 70 students now follow the programme through open

routes and this figure will most likely rise to 100 students in the third year of operation. Flexibility, however, was found to generate complexity which, ironically to some extent, requires a comparable level of bureaucracy. A dedicated MIS system to map student choice, progress and credit, was designed and tested during the first year of the programme and is now wholly operational and wholly essential.

REFERENCES

ACSTT (Advisory Committee on the Supply and Training of Teachers) (1978) Training – The Second (Haycocks) Report of the Advisory Committee on the Supply and Training of Teachers (later reformed as ACSET), HMSO, London.

Butterworth, C. (1992) More than one bite at the APEL – contrasting models of accrediting prior learning. *Journal of Further and Higher Education,* **16**(3).

Butterworth, C. and Bloor, M. (1990) Accrediting prior learning on in-service education courses for teachers, in *Realising Human Potential*, Aspects of Educational Technology 24, Kogan Page, London.

Eraut, M. (1990) Identifying the knowledge which underpins performance, in *Knowledge and Competence,* (ed. H. Black and A. Wolf), HMSO, London.

Hall, D. (1991) Credit where it's due: a flexible model. INSET by credit accumulation at Thames Polytechnic. *NASD Journal,* **25**, 40–45.

Schon, D. (1991) *The Reflective Practitioner*, 2nd edn, Avebury, London.

The position of the corporate college | 6

Bill Bailey and John Humphreys

Editors' introduction

This chapter begins an analysis of the nature and implications of the new market for education, which constitutes most of the second half of the book.

By examining three 'key transactions' of colleges, namely money, students and trained personnel, the chapter shows how the conventional 'in-house' training of the conventional DHA college is being superseded by a market situation in which both the college and the college's primary clients (NHS trusts) are corporate organizations.

A comparison of the position of colleges of health care studies with institutions of further and higher education in England and Wales is used to show that colleges are moving from unusually secure positions within health districts to uniquely exposed positions in which their future solvency is increasingly dependent on small numbers of similar and powerful employer organizations.

INTRODUCTION

Changes of status, management, resourcing and curriculum are currently affecting schools of nursing and midwifery. Institutions of further education and higher education are also experiencing changes in these areas – mainly as a consequence of the Further and Higher Education Act 1992. This chapter compares these changes with the intention of identifying the principal similarities and differences, in particular drawing out the important implications for those involved in health care education.

In its intention and implementation Project 2000 has constituted a major change in the education of nurses. The linkages the colleges have established with higher education institutions and the opportunities presented by the supernumerary status of students have enabled course teams to develop new programmes for those intending to nurse. However, these educational developments, seen by the nurse educators as central in the discussion and development of new Project 2000 courses, have now been superseded by the government's continued measures aimed at establishment of a 'market' in the National Health Service. A part of this further development has been the introduction of a market in the provision of education and training for health care workers. It will be argued that this second wave of changes will affect the working of schools of nursing (faculties of health care studies) more radically than the first period of curriculum development.

THE TRADITION

Historically, health care education and training has been the task of the schools and colleges which have been one part of a larger organization (the 'District') and providing professional and training services for that organization. This has taken the form of relatively small units enjoying a stable and secure position within the 'parent' organization, the District Health Authority (DHA). These schools and colleges have been perforce largely monotechnic institutions. The fact that, in some cases, districts have shared schools or colleges did not significantly alter this familiar model of organization. Figure 6.1(a) represents this situation where the district health authority owns and resources its college. In this, all the important movements, or transactions – of money, trainees and trained personnel – are internal ones. What is more, all the staff involved, managers, tutors and trainees, are employees of the district health authority. In these circumstances the college was an important part of its larger organization; it had no separate, legal existence, a feature important to those negotiating the merging of colleges into higher education institutions.

It is illuminating to contrast this traditional form of organization with that found in public sector further and higher education in England and Wales prior to the Education Act 1988. Figure 6.1(b) shows the position then of further education colleges and polytechnics. Like colleges of health care studies they effectively formed part of a larger organization, in this case that of the local education authority (LEA). Typically, their costs formed a relatively small part of a large total budget. As in the case of colleges of health care studies the assets (buildings and equipment) were owned and the staff were employed by the parent organization. At this point a difference emerges, since only money moved within the organization – from the LEA to the college or polytechnic. Although there were complexities in the organization of both types of institution – those providing further and higher education (FHE) and the health care institutions – the basic financial reality for both was that their main source (or

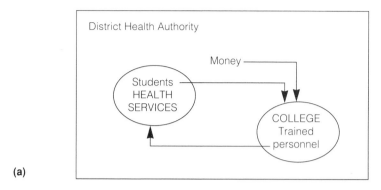

(a)

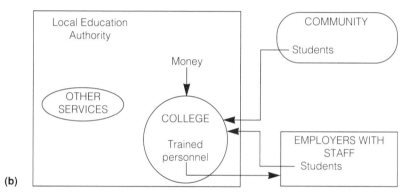

(b)

Figure 6.1 Comparison of the position of colleges of health care education and colleges of further education prior to reorganization of the two sectors. Square boxes represent self-contained 'corporate' organizations whereas ovals and circles represent groups with no legal independent status. Arrows indicate the educational relation between organizations and groups with regard to the three 'key transactions' of money, students and trained personnel. **(a)** shows the position of colleges of health care education prior to NHS reorganization and **(b)** shows the position of colleges of further education prior to their reorganization in April 1993 (at that time, polytechnics were in a similar position to further education colleges).

supply) of resource was the large 'authority', the LEA or the DHA, to which they literally belonged.

This is not to suggest that all financial resources for FHE institutions were raised locally. Some monies were raised in the form of locally levied rates but a large proportion were distributed by central government in the form of the rate support grant. There were differences in the system of aid to further education colleges and polytechnics. Resources for distribution by district health authorities to colleges of nursing derived from funds from the Department of Health.

We do not suggest that this state of affairs necessarily represented stability for the two kinds of institution and their staff. They were, for example, both subject in some cases to amalgamation and difficulties caused by cuts in resources because of the LEA's or DHA's budget problems. Also, the principals of the institutions could be heard protesting about the restrictions on their activities which they saw as deriving from their low status as the creature of larger organizations or systems. In general, though, Figure 6.1 summarizes circumstances which in certain ways benefited the two kinds of institution. Both LEAs and DHAs saw it as to their advantage to support their colleges, to keep their staffs usefully employed; and they took some pride in the development of 'their' institutions. Certainly, they did not seek to create situations that would lead to staff redundancies or redeployment, and the financial costs and loss of morale to which these would lead. There is, however, an important difference to be identified between the two sets of institutions. While further education colleges and polytechnics have always depended on attracting enough (usually, more) students each year, across a wide range of specialist areas, colleges of health care education have been dependent on a single industry.

As was stated earlier, the colleges of nursing can be seen as monotechnics having a clearly articulated relationship with their parent organization, the DHA, which in turn is the employer of their output of trained and qualified personnel. They are dependent on these in a number of important senses – for resources, for placements and for the employment of their successful trainees. The colleges in the further and higher education sector are not dependent in this way, for two important reasons. Firstly they draw students from the community at large in which the demand for courses continues to grow. Funding policies in the past have generally encouraged these institutions to recruit more students; this has been done through a reflection in its annual budget of increases in student numbers achieved by the college during the previous year. This growth has been possible because further and higher education colleges are polytechnic institutions. In turn this means that, as demand for courses, from employers or from students, has changed, they have been able to adapt their provision to that demand. In further education colleges this can be shown in the growth of GCSE and GCE A Level enrolments as vocational departments have shrunk as the result of the decline of industry during recession. This sort of response is not open to colleges of nursing whose work is dependent on a much more restricted client group. The polytechnics have similarly expanded during the last decade in response to demand from increased numbers of qualified school-leavers and adults – notably in faculties of humanities, social sciences and business studies. In brief, the public FHE colleges have always existed in a complex market situation. This is in strong contrast with the historical situation of the colleges of nursing. Furthermore, in the context of limited opportunities for re-emphasis or diversification, colleges of health care education are being exposed to competitive contracting-funding directly with the monopoly purchasers of their service. This constitutes a situation which has never been faced by public sector colleges.

While it appears to be difficult to find any parallel for the security (indicated by the key transactions in Figure 6.1(a)) enjoyed until recently by the health care colleges, it will be argued below that, in the new market environment that the government seems determined to impose on the health service, the colleges/faculties of health care studies will be confronted by more challenging circumstances than those experienced in 'mainstream' further and higher education.

THE INDEPENDENT FUTURE

Although the future of colleges of health care studies may take one of several forms, the implementation of Project 2000 has led to circumstances in which, for most colleges, the future lies within large independent corporate organizations whose business is higher education. The essence of a corporation is its separate legal existence which enables it to enter into contracts with other organizations. The corporation bears responsibility for the efficient and legal conduct of the institution's affairs and is legally empowered to act as if it is an individual person. Like other, more familiar, corporate bodies, higher education corporations own their assets (buildings, land), employ their staff and can accumulate cash reserves. They can prosper or they can fail.

During the last few years the public sectors of first, higher education, and then further education, have been 'incorporated'. In the case of the polytechnics and colleges of higher education this change followed the passing of the Education Act 1988. This Act removed the polytechnics and other colleges whose main work was higher education from their local authorities and set up a Polytechnic and Colleges Funding Council (PCFC) which took over responsibility for the planning and financing of public sector higher education. For the 'old' universities the Universities Funding Council (UFC) was formed with a constitution and role similar to those of the PCFC with respect to its institutions. The aim and effect of these decisions was to reduce the influence of local education authorities (Maclure, 1989). The Government believed that, if decisions on the allocation of courses and resources were taken nationally, the institutions, 'freed' from their local education authorities, would become more businesslike and enterprising and so would take up opportunities presented by the funding council and the world of industry and commerce. The Further and Higher Education Act 1992 rationalized the situation in higher education by creating two Higher Education Funding Councils, one each for England and Wales, which replaced the UFC and the PCFC. Also, the polytechnics and some colleges of higher education became universities.

The 1992 Act was important also for the statutory decision to remove the further education colleges from their local authorities and to give them the same corporate status as had been given to the polytechnics after 1988. Again a new national funding council was established, the Further Education Funding Council (FEFC). This Council (itself incorporated) is charged with a broad remit: principally, to assist the colleges in raising participation rates of 16–18-year-olds and to promote the quality of further education programmes as they contribute to the achievement of National Education and Training Targets. The FEFC supported the Colleges as they prepared for their new corporate status which they assumed on 1 April 1993. Their position with regard to the transactions we have identified can be represented as in Figure 6.2(a). That position is, given the historical diversity of the further education sector, more complex than that of the universities – or of health care colleges. While the bulk of the funding for

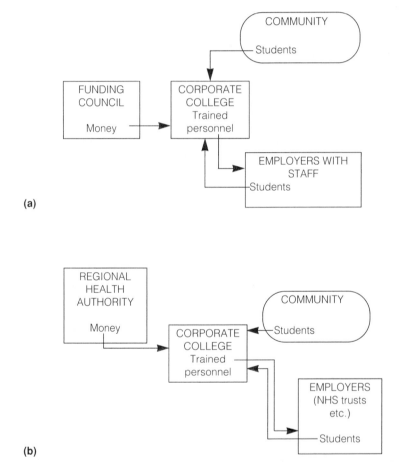

Figure 6.2 Comparison of the positions of colleges of further educations and universities with colleges of health care education after reorganization of the two sectors. Square boxes represent corporate organizations, whereas ovals or circles represent groups with no legal independent status. Arrows indicate the educational relationship with regard to the three key transactions of money, students and trained personnel. **(a)** shows the position of further education colleges and universities and **(b)** shows the position of colleges of health care studies.

further education colleges comes via the FEFC (out of money previously spent by LEAs on their colleges), there are other sources of finance. The chief of these are the Training and Enterprise Councils (TECs) which agree (i.e. contract for) the provision of some work-related courses in colleges, as well as Youth Training and Employment Training programmes. Some colleges receive finance from the European Social Fund (ESF) for agreed projects and many put on 'full cost' tailor-made courses for local companies and organizations. Additionally, it should be recorded that the FEFC in the first year of its existence took on responsibility for the allocation of PICKUP funds (for professional and industrial updating) and for ACCESS funds to further education colleges.

In summary, the years since 1988 have seen radical changes in the organization and funding of public sector higher and further education institutions in England and Wales. Each institution now operates as a corporation and is independent in the sense that it is in charge of its operations and can make decisions about its use of its resources, physical, financial and human. Colleges and the universities now receive their allocation of funds from national councils which distribute the government's allocations of monies for FHE according to (changing) methodologies based on views of national 'needs' and to some degree on an assessment of the quality and efficiency of the service provided by the institutions. In 1993, for example, the HEFC for England decided to reduce funding for students on arts and humanities programmes in an attempt to steer institutions towards more vocationally useful science and technology courses. The FEFC, on the other hand, is still, at the time of writing, consulting with the colleges on a new funding methodology. What is clear is that it will not be a simple allocation based on 'entry', i.e. based on numbers enrolled on courses and programmes. It will reflect colleges' abilities to retain students 'on course' and the achievements of students at the point of 'exit' (their accreditation by examining and validating bodies). Both the further and higher education sectors have seen significant increases in student numbers over the last five years – despite the decline in the size of the age groups caused by demographic factors, but also the result in part of the economic recession. A significant proportion of this expansion has been achieved by increased efficiency rather than new money.

Although there are alternatives, present evidence suggests that most colleges of health care studies will be incorporated into large higher education corporations: that is, into 'old' or 'new' universities. In these circumstances, their position as far as important transactions and movements of resources and students are concerned will be very much the same for the purposes of this comparison. Figure 6.2(b) shows the position of colleges as they separate from the district health authorities. Since the DHAs have no longer any direct role in education and training they are omitted from this figure. It will be seen that all the key transactions now involve interaction with bodies or institutions external to the college. Students are/will be recruited from the community at large and enrolled as supernumerary pre-registration nurses on Project 2000 courses or they will come from NHS trusts, which will also be the future employers of newly trained personnel. The situation in which the college is placed is that of a market, in which it will have to compete with other similar organizations to obtain contracts. Its success in obtaining such contracts for initial and post-initial training will determine its solvency and, therefore, its survival. In this market situation, no health service organization (RHA or DHA) is financially responsible for protecting a college if it fails to secure funding by contracts. This will be the case even if the college forms a faculty of a university, since the university will be reluctant to use what are likely to be limited cash reserves to subsidize loss-making operations. Also, both the internal politics and auditing procedures of the universities will be likely to prevent funding council allocations for students on other programmes being transferred to ailing health care faculties.

In this new era the unique situation of the health care faculties is likely to become clear. Unlike the corporate further education colleges and universities generally, who are working to national funding councils which are charged to increase numbers of students on courses, the reorganized health care faculties will depend for their future funding on contracts competitively allocated by a limited number of service providers. The role of the RHAs in relation to Working Paper 10 (WP10) is to spend to ensure 'regional self-sufficiency' in terms of the supply of trained personnel and their in-service training. There is no reason why regional health authorities should recognize traditional DHA boundaries by contracting with the college which has historically provided training for a DMU or NHS trust. We can extend this argument and speculate that, provided adequate and good quality training is offered, the regions could contract with successful colleges outside their area. These could, for example, provide some of the training by means of distance learning methods and, for direct teaching purposes, lease local premises.

In this competitive climate, the colleges/faculties will be scrutinized for quality and cost-effectiveness in ways they have not experienced hitherto. Furthermore, as purchasers of education become increasingly aware that they are spending resources on behalf of service-providers, a situation without precedent in professional or vocational education is likely to emerge. In Figure 6.3 we represent the situation where RHAs establish consortia of service providers to make decisions on contracts for education and training.

In these circumstances, although WP10 moneys technically flow from the RHA to the colleges, the consortia make the contract decisions. It is they, the consortia, which have effective control of the colleges' money supply and, therefore, their solvency. It can be seen that the key transactions, again of money, students and trained personnel, take place between a college and the service providers with whom it is contracted to provide training. Since they become effectively the direct purchasers and receivers of training, the consortia are (or will be) critically important clients uniquely positioned to determine a college's future. While some RHAs may intend to secure colleges during a period of transition, in order to give them time to adapt to the new context,

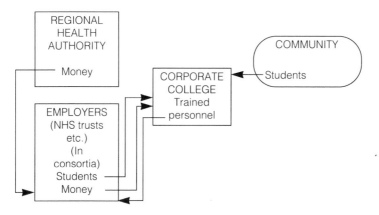

Figure 6.3 The position of colleges of health care education where regional health authorities delegate control of education contracting to consortia of NHS trusts. The diagram is technically inaccurate in that, since consortia have no legal standing, education funding must flow direct from region to colleges or via one trust acting as agent for the consortium. However the presentation of money flow via the consortia gives a more accurate impression of the importance of trusts as clients of corporate colleges/faculties. It is argued in the text that there is no precedent for this situation in post-compulsory education and training.

others will not. Already in some regions all education and training contracts are nationally advertised and open to tender. To have a long-term future in these conditions, we suggest that colleges will need to change radically their approaches to curriculum and institutional development.

It is our view that the situation shown in Figure 6.3 is new and unique in that the solvency and survival of a college could be decided by the award of a single contract by a small number of large employers. For this we can find no parallel in British post-compulsory education and training. In the public sectors of further and higher education the national funding councils are guaranteeing – in the interests of the stability of institutions – substantial core funding. Typically this core forms 90% of the previous year's funding and the remainder ('marginal funding') is available on the basis of institutions' bids and/or awards on the basis of measures of quality and efficiency. For the health care colleges and faculties a key factor will be the extent to which RHAs decide to give colleges a degree of protection by intervening if employers' consortia are inclined, intentionally or otherwise, effectively to close a college by the non-award of a contract (even a 10% loss of funding could be sufficient to render a college insolvent). It may be that this form of protection will be necessary to encourage university corporations to take on the commitment to substantial numbers of staff for whom redundancy costs in the event of reduction and closure would be high. It seems highly unlikely that all RHAs will adopt such a protective policy and none will do so indefinitely.

It has been argued elsewhere that the health care faculties and colleges will, if they are to survive in the conditions created by the imposition of the 'training market', have to adopt a marketing approach to their work (Humphreys, 1993). This will require them to switch from the patient-as-client as their primary curriculum and professional focus. This was acceptable and, indeed, appropriate in the traditional in-house model (Figure 6.1(a)), but in the emerging context they will need to address their thinking to a new client – the service-provider. This shift will be for most colleges a contentious and difficult matter, and it lies at the very heart of the radically new situation they are facing. In the first place the nature and the quality of their provision of education and training will be assessed against the needs of their clients. As these clients, the service providers, influence or take control of education contracts, they are almost certainly going to increase the accuracy and force of their articulation of needs and requirements. It will be in the context of contract negotiation that service priorities, the trainees' personal and professional development and the needs of the patients can be educationally reconciled.

Thus, programmes of education and training will be designed in the strategic as well as the professional context. They will be purchased, and therefore viewed increasingly, as a key part of a coherent strategy of institutional and staff development, possibly linked to IPR. The role of the nurse tutor will change more profoundly than has been necessary so far in the implementation of Project 2000 courses. From 'guardians of the profession', nurse tutors will become education and training professionals working constructively with their clients, service provider managers and staff. This change of emphasis will lead to conflict as the differences between provision based on needs identified by clients and those identified by professional groups become apparent. At this point the reaction and response of colleges will be critical and the future will be in the hands of the nurse-tutor curriculum development teams. The risk must be that, in the absence of a suitable model of curriculum development (and, of course, for most tutors, of any experience of working for client organizations of the new kind), staff will withdraw into an orthodoxy of commitment to the profession rather than accept the reality of commitment to the client. Commitment to the profession, a manifestation of traditional view of the patient-as-client, might thus be seen as a means of avoiding the necessity of acknowledging the strategic needs and increasingly self-confident demands of service provider organizations. It would also prevent a start being made on the difficult but creative engagement in the task of reconciling issues of quality and relevance as defined by clients, with definitions of these as defined by the National Boards for Nursing, Midwifery and Health Visiting or by the academic standards committees of universities. The design of programmes for education and training cannot be undertaken by the nurse tutor, or course teams, in isolation. Many – if not all – aspects of the college's organization will influence the adaptation to the new ways of working. In particular institutional structure will need to be changed to 'mirror' client organizations so that information on needs (for design) and evaluation (for responsive teaching and training) can flow in both directions.

With the forthcoming demise of regional health authorities, the future mechanism for education remains unclear. However it is unlikely that the ascendancy of the NHS trust or the incorporation of colleges will be reversed. Therefore, the position of colleges/faculties will remain essentially similar to that described above. In these circumstances, institutional development will need to facilitate curriculum and staff development if attempts to respond to the new clients are not to be frustrated by bureaucracy. There is much to be done.

REFERENCES

Humphreys, J. (1993) The marketing gap in health care education. *Nurse Education Today*, **13**, 202–209.

Maclure, S. (1989) *Education Reformed*, Hodder & Stoughton, London.

The market for education: supply and demand

Stephanie Stanwick

Editors' introduction

If, as asserted in Chapter 6, NHS trusts are the primary clients of colleges, then their position must be properly understood. This chapter begins with a review of the purpose and nature of NHS reorganization and uses this to identify current issues for NHS trusts. The author draws out some implications, particularly with regard to quantitative and qualitative aspects of the demand for education.

INTRODUCTION

Many people in nurse education today, if asked, would state that their *raison d'être* was to provide good quality nursing care through the education they provide to nurses who pass through their establishments, the argument being that well educated nurses are better equipped to deliver that quality of care to patients. It is probably safe to say that, although educationalists have added to the list of skills deemed necessary for the modern nurse to work in today's environment, there have been few developments in preparing nurses to work within the new organizations and their environments in the managed market of health care today, and in particular the independent hospitals and community health care trusts. In fact one could be forgiven for assuming, from much that is written in the professional journals, that such a market environment was the antithesis of all that was held dear by the professional nurse and those who contribute to her/his education. Most individuals who look for courses that examine health care delivery in a business environment and thereby help to develop the required knowledge and skills to work in such a situation would not think of post-registration schools of nursing and midwifery education as the starting point in their search for such relevant courses, and neither would their managers. There must therefore be a considerable gap between preparing an individual to practise on the one hand, whether at a pre-registration or a post-registration level, and preparing that individual to practise in today's organizational environment on the other.

In the consumer-orientated world of competitive markets, the fitness for its purpose of a product goes beyond simple assessments of technical performance. Additional assessments of satisfactory performance must be made in the context of the environment within which the product will function. As an analogy, the Mini is a very appropriate car to own in the city – technically it is well suited to that situation, parking is easy and petrol consumption is good – but it would not be your vehicle of choice if you were about to undertake an expedition into rough mountain terrain. This would be even more true should that expedition have a competitive edge to it so that there was a significant bonus in finishing first. A Land Rover might be more fit for that purpose. Although both cars have engines that work, that propel the wheels round and enable people to travel from A to B, it is obvious that one is more appropriate than the other in each of the situations described. If you use that analogy in education then one could argue that without the relevant preparation for practice today – which also takes into account the situation that practitioners may find themselves in, over and above that face-to-face patient contact – then the 'product of education', i.e. the practitioner, will never be completely fit for the purpose.

You could apply fitness for purpose in pre-registration education in relation to the hospital trust's business of dealing with faster-turnover, shorter-length-of-stay, higher-dependency patients, and consider whether current education really does prepare the student for that environment. Although one expects pre-registration education to lay the foundations for continued professional education, that foundation itself must be appropriate, otherwise considerable time effort and money will be spent after qualifying in trying to provide practitioners with the skills that could easily have been provided earlier.

Up until quite recently, colleges of nursing and midwifery education have by and large been spectators in the recent NHS reforms, and have watched from the sidelines with considerable interest to see what was happening to their clinical colleagues. However, many now realize that colleges of health care education are no longer immune from the purchaser/provider split and the effects of the managed market for health care services, and in reality many have been pulled well and truly into that arena over the past couple of years. The pace of that change has varied. In many parts of the country colleges are just beginning to realize that they too are going to be deeply affected by these organizational changes, while today's truth has been with others for some considerable time.

THE PURCHASER/PROVIDER SPLIT IN HEALTH CARE SERVICES

NHS reform stems from the three White Papers: *Promoting Better Health*, *Working for Patients* and *Caring for People* (Department of Health, 1987; 1989a; b). These were designed to tackle the underlying problems of management and funding in the health services. The objective was to bring an 'internal' market element into resource allocation processes which were previously dominated by planning and line management hierarchies. Through the introduction of these far reaching reforms the various elements of the NHS were expected to behave more competitively within a market-like framework, to reduce costs and respond to incentives for efficiency, performance and quality. The most important aspects of the reforms introduced:

1. a system of contractual funding;
2. proposals to strengthen management at all levels;
3. new arrangements for allocating resources;
4. measures to manage clinical activity;
5. measures to improve the quality and efficiency of services;
6. ways of reinforcing the importance of the community as the focus for the provision for services.

In this scenario the traditional role of the district health authority (DHA) changed; to them was attributed the role of purchasers or commissioners of health services responsible for contracting for appropriate health care services for their resident populations with a wide ranging number of service providers. As every successive 'wave' of hospital and community trusts came on line, the DHAs saw their old-style 'management units' being transformed into these new independent organizations who were accountable to their local populations for the services they provided and directly accountable to the management executive of the NHS (NHSME) via the NHSME 'Outposts' for their financial probity.

There were many who argued in the early days of the reforms that these organizational changes would not of themselves be sufficient to introduce a market element into health care provision. Perhaps there was a little bit of wishful thinking in all of this, for the pace of the change for many was so quick there was a very real 'culture shock'. These people hoped that the market itself would end up being a figment of everyone's imagination – never actually materializing – and though funding mechanisms through contracting might change, the status quo in respect of current patterns of service delivery would somehow be maintained. However for most the market for health care became very real and created very real business and professional dilemmas very quickly.

With the speed of implementation of the NHS reforms in some DHAs, colleges were left, in respect of both their management structure and their accountability, a little at odds with the changing face of provider reorganizations. Previously many directors of nurse education had reported to the chief nurse of the DHA, but after the first and second wave of trust implementation the traditional chief nurse's role was obsolete. Many left, choosing to become the executive nurses of these trusts, while others took on a corporate role for quality and standards within the purchasing arena. In either case the organizational structure of colleges became inappropriate in several ways: firstly, in that representatives from the health services had 'seats' at the council table or management board of the colleges; and secondly in the colleges' arrangements for their management and financial accountability. It raised the question that some had already anticipated and begun to debate: where should colleges of education sit in the purchaser provider split of health services? The answer for many colleges was that they should be integrated into and with institutes of higher education, albeit in a variety of different ways, and to such effect that they fell outside the perceived remit of the NHS.

The 'demand' for education, both in respect of the type of activity and its volume, will be driven by the hospital and community trusts to a great extent, and therefore one must begin to understand some of the dilemmas that the trusts face before exploring how that will impact on education.

Most people working in the health services today realize that the concept of the market for health care is not synonymous with a true industrial, 'for-profits' market model. Indeed the health care market has been described variously as a managed market, an internal market, a regulated managed market structure and an implied internal market. Debate has tended to focus on the more extreme competitive version of the market; however von Otter (1991) suggests that the competitive influence in health care provision is aimed at securing greater internal efficiency of provider organizations, greater responsiveness of service provision to patients' preferences and increased managerial effectiveness.

Salter (1991) maintains that the internal market set out to control demand by means of the commissioning process, and similarly Heginbotham (1992) describes rationing and priority setting as the central issue to purchasing dilemmas (for example the issue of 'acute' versus community care, or the issue of equity between all care groups versus priorities within those care groups). All agree that the potential for increased demand and costs for health care is unlimited.

One clear expression of the market has been the speed with which referrals into the London hospitals for some specialist services began to fall. Butler and Millar (1992), reporting on the problems facing University College and Middlesex Hospitals, surmised that once the brakes had been taken off no one expected the internal market to 'scuttle away with the speed it has'. These London hospitals expected a 15–20% decrease in activity from distant purchasing authorities but in reality some experienced a decrease in referrals in some specialties of up to 71% in one year. The Kings Fund Commission 1992, *London Health Care 2010*, made radical recommendations for changes in service provision in London, advocating a system of hospital closures, a reduction in acute beds and an increase in community-based services for the capital. Similar issues were addressed in the Tomlinson report (1992), *Report of the*

Inquiry into London Health Service, and by the more recent report (Department of Health, 1993) *Making London Better* and the recently published review of specialties. Whichever way you look at it, triggered by the internal market or not, we are going to see radical changes in service delivery in the immediate future.

Some argue that the general practitioner fundholding scheme (GPFH) was established to 'kick-start' the market, and a recent study into GPFH undertaken by the London School of Economics, reported by Robinson *et al.* (1992), describes how fundholders have begun to exercise 'exit rights' where problems have been identified on waiting lists or where patients express preferences for treatment. This means that where GPFHs have negotiated their own contracts for services with hospital and community providers they have, in many cases, chosen not to support the traditional patterns of services in, or referrals to their local providers, choosing rather to place contracts elsewhere on the grounds of quality.

All these issues have combined to make health care provision for some trusts a very risky business with the result that current service provision, changing and new service developments will all be scrutinized very carefully by the Trusts, their chief executives and their boards. There will be a constant reappraisal of 'what is done' and 'the way it is done' in order to deliver the cost and quality improvements demanded by purchasers and GPFHs alike.

THE MARKET FOR EDUCATION

The implementation of the NHS and Community Care Act 1990 brought radical changes not only in the way hospital and community health services were organized but also in the way nursing, midwifery, health visiting, paramedical and scientific education and training was to be funded. The system suggested and implemented through Working Paper 10 (WP10) was complex to understand and to implement, but it demanded a fundamental separation of key aspects of educational funding from the contractual funding of health services generally. To be understood fully one has to understand that funding for education was complicated anyway. Before the reforms funding for nursing, midwifery and health visiting education came from a variety of sources; from the English National Board for some aspects of pre-registration education, (though student salaries were part of DHA resources); from centrally funded initiatives e.g. for 'Hi-tech' training, and directly from the Department of Health for Project 2000 implementation. One must not forget also that many initiatives in post-registration nursing education came from 'soft monies' as year on year many chief nurses found vacancy monies that could be diverted to fund developments in education. This meant that significant amounts of money for education was found not in formally described education and training budgets but in the savings made in other places, such as staff budgets, and so in many instances the money for developments was found from creative budgeting. When faced with the regional requirements in the base year of WP10 implementation, to quantify and ring-fence the resources used to support education and training of nurses, midwives and health visitors, much of that money proved to be so entwined with DHA resources that most regional health authorities (RHAs) spent the next two years trying to equate training activity with money. What happened in practice was that many district finance officers, when asked to identify education monies in line with the WP10 principles in readiness for regional 'top slicing' or ring-fencing, could only go to the formal education budgets and significant proportions of the total resource spent was therefore missing, making the process of marrying up total education activity with the required resource very difficult.

The principles of Working Paper 10 funding and its relationship to the newly introduced contractual funding for health care were twofold: firstly to protect education during the early years of the internal market when education might be susceptible to cuts , and secondly to enable fairer price comparisons for services between different hospitals and between different community health services. Provider units who were great 'supporters' of education, for example those who had large schools of pre-registration nursing and midwifery education and post registration education, might, in a service price comparison with provider units who had no such education service to support on site, be placed at a considerable disadvantage. The argument was that the cost and price of a replacement hip operation in hospital A would be higher than hospital B because A had high education costs. In such a scenario education might be vulnerable as provider unit A sought to reduce its costs in line with provider unit B. By removing the resources for education from that arena it enabled a more equitable comparison of service prices.

The details of Working Paper 10 funding became more complicated when looking at how a traditional pre-registration student's salary should be treated. It was argued that a traditional student gave considerable 'hands-on' care to patients in hospital settings during her training, and approximately 60% of her/his time was spent as an integral part of the rostered ward team, and that therefore that proportion of her/his salary should rightly stay with hospitals and trusts and be reflected within their service prices while the remaining 40%, which was considered as 'education' should be included in the ring-fenced money. There were similar splits for most courses and only a few student salaries fell into the 100% ring-fenced category. Table 7.1 shows the split between ring-fenced education monies and those that were not ring-fenced and remained with hospital and community trusts.

The ring-fenced 'pot' of money enabled a 'purchaser/provider split' to be introduced within education. That money was held by the RHAs who became the 'purchasers' of education, while the colleges of health care studies became the 'providers'. The purchaser/provider split in education has many similarities to that within health care services in that:

1. a system of contracts and contractual funding was introduced between the RHA and the providers of education;

Table 7.1   Ring-fenced and non-ring-fenced education monies

Ring fenced	Non-ring-fenced
Tutor salaries	60% pre-registration student salaries
Course costs	A percentage of the following salaries and bursaries: enrolled nurses' conversion, midwifery students, Project 2000
Costs for certain services – telephone cleaning, etc.	
Project 2000 implementation costs	
A percentage of pre-registration student bursaries salaries, enrolled nurses, conversion salaries, Project 2000 bursaries and midwifery student salaries and bursaries	Post-registration student salaries
100% DN, HN, CPN student salaries	

2. the RHA commissioning education according to the needs of its 'population' translates into the needs of the hospital and community services for appropriately trained staff;
3. there is a managed competition or market between providers of education;
4. the process of contracting draws attention to issues of cost-efficiency and quality within education services.

Figure 7.1 sets out broadly the relationship between RHA, Trusts and colleges.

However one must add that the processes are not similar in every detail in every region in England. The RHAs were given the task of implementing WP10 in line with certain key principles but the details varied in the various regions.

In examining the principles of an internal market for education we can now see reflected those characteristics of the internal market for health care described earlier. In summary, von Otter (1991) thought that the market would bring about greater efficiency, greater responsiveness with greater managerial effectiveness. Salter's (1991) view was that the market was a way of controlling demand, and Heginbotham (1992) thought that it would enable rationing and priority setting.

All these characteristics can also be applied to the market for education and the remainder of this chapter will be devoted to examining these issues in some detail.

THE DEMAND FOR EDUCATION

The 'demand' for education has two aspects: first, the numbers required for courses and second, the type and content of those courses. From a college's point of view the demand for the course concerns the number of appropriate students who can be attracted to join a course in order to make it viable in respect of the investment in time and resources that the college will put into it.

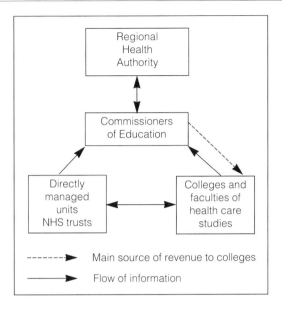

Figure 7.1 Simplified relationships of the purchaser/provider split in education (from Humphreys, 1993)

From a trust's point of view, however, demand for the course concerns how many appropriately qualified people will be available to work at the end of it.

Therefore there are two aspects of 'demand', numbers of people and skills they have gained. From a trust's perspective the demand for education may more appropriately be described as part of its overall workforce supply issues. From the RHA's point of view 'demand' has yet another flavour in that the region is concerned about numbers of appropriately skilled staff within its total geographical area, and for all its health care services and specialties. Qualified people may go and work in the region next door, and qualified people from that region may come and work in the first region and providing these numbers broadly cancel each other out then the region satisfies its demand for training and is 'self-sufficient'. The RHA's view of demand is therefore about self-sufficiency in education and training for its own hospitals and community health services. However it must be noted that broad self-sufficiency on a regional level can mask considerable local variations and difficulties. These will become more apparent as the factors affecting an individual trust's demand are discussed in more detail.

One could argue from a historical perspective, and with some justification, that the NHS overall has never got its demand right, and that looking back there has either been a feast or a famine. Conroy and Stidson (1988) anticipated what they described as 'the black hole', a term used to highlight the considerable problems for the NHS workforce caused by demographic changes and shortages in the labour market. These included a reduction in the number of school leavers; increased competitiveness of the part-time labour market; the age structure of the population and the reduction in unemployment levels. They went on to predict a very real 'crisis' for the NHS in the 1990s. Yet well into the 1990s new qualifiers are still not able to find jobs and large numbers of applications are received for many jobs that are advertised. It would be easy to say that there are no problems, but again the global picture masks very real specific problems, for example nationally there is a shortage of paediatric nurses, specialist ITU nurses and CPNs.

'Top-down' approaches to 'demand', as used by RHAs and the Department of Health rely largely on being able to predict nursing staff turnover. Cavanagh (1989) identified the problem that 'turnover' in nursing affected both the cost and the quality of care. Cavanagh (1990) went on to try and identify 'predictors' of turnover from both the literature and research but due to the variables involved was not able to draw conclusions. This inevitably leads us to question the reliability of using 'turnover' as an indicator within these 'top-down' approaches to quantifying demand.

WP10 places responsibility for determining demand for education squarely at the door of the trusts. In other words the demand for education must relate to and be driven by the workforce supply needs of trusts, with the RHAs having a say from their perspective of 'self-sufficiency'. If this is achieved then perhaps there will be a marriage of 'top-down' with 'bottom-up' approaches that could achieve greater success in the numbers game than has previously been achieved.

As has been discussed earlier there must be a large element of appropriate skills analysis in the 'demand' equation. From a Trust's point of view, if they are to survive in the competitive environment (where GPFHs withdraw their contracts for services with local hospitals and community services on the grounds of quality) then the issue of staff and skills will become fundamental. Many educationalists argue that trusts do not know what they want in respect of staff and skills, and this may well be the case for some; however, if this is true then it presents an exciting opportunity for those colleges articulate enough to talk to trusts about their future business, provided they have staff with the skills needed to deliver that service.

At this point in time probably the best that can be anticipated is that colleges, using Moss Kanter's (1989) descriptions for corporations must be: 'Fast, Flexible, Focused and Friendly'. In other words, colleges must respond quickly to the needs of trusts, they must be flexible in how and where they are prepared to put on courses; these courses must be focused enough to deliver not only a nationally recognized qualification for the practitioner but local needs and variations as well; and lastly, relationships between the two parties must be friendly. Both should enjoy doing business with each other. Stanwick (1993) argues that both nurses and nursing in the future need to 'learn how to dance', they will need to deal with new roles in new settings; they will be led by a new kind of manager who thrives in a changing and challenging environment; they will need to lead innovation and demonstrate imagination and they will need educational programmes that are both flexible and cost-effective to provide the skills and knowledge for the practitioners of the future.

The nursing profession has not, by and large, been noted for its flexibility of approach and in fact many would argue that it has been rigid and narrow. However new roles and flexibility of working are going to be central to nursing in the future. There has for a long time been a 'substitution' of tasks between different grades and qualifications of staff. For instance the DHSS (1986) in their review of skill mix found that staff skills available on wards on a day-to-day, week-to-week basis varied enormously; this was also found by the Audit Commission (1991). It could therefore be concluded that what was appropriate for one nurse to do one day becomes inappropriate on the next as a more senior nurse is on duty. Most nurses are familiar with the situation that exists for many enrolled nurses. When it is appropriate they are left in charge of wards and may well be responsible for administering intravenous drugs but the next day, when the staff nurse is back on duty, they are given less 'responsible' work. Even within the primary nursing model of care, the role of enrolled nurses as associate nurse is blurred. So it would appear that an element of role flexibility already exists when the need arises. Surely the ideal way would be to plan for such flexibility, developing roles, providing the added knowledge and skills through education and evaluating the effectiveness of these roles formally.

The Department of Health (1989c) has for some time recognized that certain tasks previously performed by doctors could be delegated to nurses, and if the recommendations made by the Ministerial Group on Junior Doctors' Hours (Department of Health, 1990) are to be met, then arguably nurses will need to accept some of the responsibilities currently undertaken by doctors. The challenge for nurses and nursing is that they grasp the opportunity presented by these issues and develop new roles in both the hospital and community that are innovative, exciting and challenging, taking on activities previously within the remit of doctors but creating something that is uniquely their own and of enormous benefit to patient care. If nurses can match up to this agenda they will contribute to the business agenda of the trusts, helping them to secure their business in a competitive environment. Colleges of health care education must therefore be leading the challenge and the innovations, helping trusts to prepare individuals in readiness for their new roles.

EDUCATION DEMAND AND WORKFORCE SUPPLY

The accurate calculation of education demand will only be achieved by structured and systematic frameworks for quantifying workforce supply issues in trusts.

As a starting point, trusts must be able to describe in great detail exactly how their workforce is currently made up. Table 7.2 sets out the sort of questions that need to be answered by each organization, and they will all be very different.

Table 7.2　A workforce profile

How many? What kind? Specialist (professional) groups
Part-time/Full-time?
How long do they stay?
Where do they live?
Where do they go when they leave?
What makes them stay?
How are roles changing?
What are the skills shortages?
What about succession planning?
Who trains them?

For example, a community-based trust in a rural area may have a very slow turnover of staff, a lot of part-time workers, mature women with families, who all travel and work locally in relation to their homes. A similar trust in an urban area may have few part-time staff, with a higher turnover rate; the age group of their workforce overall may be younger, with fewer mature women supporting families. The first trust may use a number of colleges for their education and training while the second may rely solely on a college serving a fairly large geographical area. These two trusts, each with a similar business, have very different workforce profiles. From such a profile the trust should be able to assess the numbers of their workforce that they traditionally recruit from training, the percentage of part-timers, turnover rates and wastage rates, and from this they can make judgements about the kind of recruitment and retention policy they will need in the future, together with the other policies that, when combined, will form the trust's workforce strategy. Each trust can then assess the impact that such policies might have on their future demand for training if the targets identified were successfully achieved.

However the picture is incomplete without reference to the context of their recruitment market. For example a trust planning to reduce its demand for education (because it was anticipating an increasing ability to recruit from a local labour pool of mature, qualified people returning to work after a break for childcare) would need to assess whether these people were there in the first place, who the competing employers were and how attractive an employment package could be offered to induce them to join the trust's workforce. Table 7.3 lists questions of relevance in a competitive labour market.

The most difficult aspect in matching or balancing 'supply' with 'demand' is working through assumptions about how one particular aspect will impact on another, and from this making a commitment to an appropriate course of action. The key, once started, is to evaluate progress frequently, to revisit the original assumptions and to see whether, in the light of new situations and new information received, the original course of action still holds good or whether there needs to be a change in emphasis.

Table 7.3   The competing labour market

Who are the competing employers?
Who are the competitive trainers?
Local pay? Benefits?
Travel to work patterns?
Number of suitable 18 year olds?
Specialist skills?
Number of mature entrants?
Number of returners?
Mobility? Unemployment?
Housing?
National shortage of skills?
National pay strategies and benefits

An example of the difficulties of matching supply and demand is well illustrated by the falling numbers of health visitor and district nursing students in training. It would be very easy to place the problem solely at the door of changing labour markets, but it is in fact more complicated. Traditionally community services have supported upwards of six such student places every year, this equating to their demand for education once their own labour market had been assessed. However these numbers have fallen quite sharply over the past few years for a variety of reasons. Firstly, the turnover rate fell amongst qualified health visiting and district nursing staff – some with families found that, instead of being the provider of a second income, due to redundancy and unemployment of their partners they were in the position of sole earner. Secondly, many community trusts evaluating the roles and skill mix of their staff found that the requirements for qualified staff then fell due to an enhancement in the roles of other staff within the community team; and thirdly, some community units looking at the training offered by many colleges found that the knowledge and skills provided by the courses were not as pertinent as they had been to the future business of the trusts.

A proportion of colleges of education have risen to the challenge, devising courses on a modular approach that a variety of staff can access as well as the student community practitioner. However some trusts have had to approach alternative education providers to provide the innovative competency-based training that the trust decided was necessary for the future of its business. This scenario has led to one college losing out to the benefit of another, because it was not prepared to 'compromise on its professional values'. One can hypothesize that, should such trends continue, there might well be a number of such colleges who find that the continuation of community courses is no longer a viable option. Alternatively, colleges currently involved in community health care education may 'diversify', finding alternative education and training needs to be met: for example where new developmental roles of staff are being tried out in community services, then colleges could step in to offer modules that bridge the gap and provide the relevant knowledge and skills.

Table 7.4 sets out some of the other internal organizational factors that have some bearing on the question of demand.

Table 7.4   Workforce change

* Reprofiling, local pay issues
* Work based training and NVQs
* Support workers
* Skill mix, grade mix
* Changing practice
* Audit standards
* Roles, Teams
* Cross functional collaboration
* Professional boundary changes

These are related to the very specific, individual and local factors of trusts, their local patterns of work, local schemes for team working and collaboration, schemes which examine the overlap between some of the professional and functional groups. All of these will have significant impact on education both in respect of the demand in numbers, i.e. 'activity' and type of course – its content and quality. In any event, it is inevitable that the pattern and volume of education cannot be fixed year on year if colleges are going to face up to the challenge of changing health care.

Inevitably the demand for education may be much easier to get right in post-registration education and training than in pre-registration training. The lead-in time and response time for curriculum change will allow colleges to respond much more quickly and more flexibly if they decide to. Indeed much of the ground work is already there with the ENB Framework and Higher award, and many colleges have already addressed the issues of similar competences required by many of the so called hi-tech courses, or the communication skills required in both mental health and care of the elderly. Many colleges are already offering a 'menu' of mix-and-match modules that individually and collectively offer the variety of educational courses that the health care provider of today requires and wants.

Pre-registration education, because of its long lead time, offers a different set of challenges. It is more difficult to predict health service changes over a four- or five-year time frame, and given the pace of change, particularly in London, with hospitals closing and merging, the demand for education is far harder to anticipate and get right. However simply because it is harder doesn't mean that it cannot be tackled in a similar systematic way. One thing is certain: trusts will always need qualified nurses; the uncertainty lies more in the subsequent specialization of those nurses at a post-registration level than in pre-registration requirements. None the less, colleges could do much more to make pre-registration education 'fit for purpose' – i.e. the business of trusts.

CHANGE – BY DEFAULT OR DESIGN

There is a cautionary tale for all involved with mental handicap nurse education (RNMH). Here many RHAs have been faced with the choice either to interfere with the market or let some courses sink without trace. The fact is that education has not kept pace with the changes in service provision and this is not because of inflexibility on the part of colleges (by and large), but because the service itself could not make up its mind what kind of practitioner it wanted to deliver the service model and its underpinning philosophy, given that much of the service was being provided in true community settings and on a multi-agency basis. To a certain extent two schools of thought emerged: the 'pro social-worker' faction on the one hand, and the 'pro nurse faction' on the other, and this was reflected by the colleges.

There have been no outright winners from this saga; however the people that come closest to it are the services and colleges that recognize that there is room for both professions' skills, and indeed where both are recognized as being necessary and are valued.

The point to be made is that, although change was required, in the vacuum of non-agreement between service providers and colleges many courses were faced with problems of viability that left commissioners of education with a choice between intervening to save the course on the grounds that what was provided was better than nothing at all, or letting the course fold because services did not seem to want to support it.

Change in education, to be successful, must be 'by design' and not 'by default' but this needs close cooperation between all players.

The change process within trusts themselves must be closely managed. The strategic direction or plan for the trust should not stop at the corporate board, but has to filter through the organization so that every manager who is in the position to commit resources on behalf of the trust 'signs up' to the strategy and change. What tends to happen is that strategic change is agreed at board level but at clinical directorate level there is little understanding of or commitment to what is proposed. This needs to be clearly understood by education staff, who may have close discussions with the senior nurse of the directorate about future needs for courses and service developments only to find that her/his views are way out of line with the view of the trust board itself, which could result in a great deal of unnecessary and unproductive work.

THE MARKET RELATIONSHIP – CHANGING PLAYERS

The relationship of the purchaser/provider split in education portrayed in Figure 7.1 is a much simplified one. The role of the RHA as the commissioner of education will change as the role of regions themselves change with the outcome of the review of the 'interim tier' – a term used by the NHSME for a level of the organization that will sit between the NHSME and commissioners of service. Many RHAs have begun to devolve part of their commissioning function for education to what are described as 'consortia of providers'. These consortia are groups of trusts who collaborate together to purchase the education that they require both in terms of activity, type and content of courses.

The identity of the future purchaser of education may be debatable, but the principle of contractual funding will not change: it will continue to be the method by which education providers are made more responsive to local providers, more cost-effective and efficient; and if contracting as a process is here to stay then a market – managed, internal or otherwise – will continue to develop. Similarly, the demand for education will be driven by trusts both in the numbers required for courses and the nature of those courses themselves, and quite simply colleges who 'deliver' will retain the business and those who do not will not. Whatever the prevailing system, that system will have to ensure that the views of the trusts are central to the whole equation; after all they employ the people and they may simply vote with their feet if their views are not taken on board.

Obviously the processes of purchasing and contracting are closely entwined, and in order to effect changes within both services, education and health care, a mature relationship between the key players, a collaborative partnership, must emerge. As in the contracting processes for health care services generally, more sophisticated forms of contracts for education will emerge over time. Such contracts will allow for the flexibility and responsiveness required for post-registration education on the one hand but give some stability to pre-registration education on the other, with greater articulation of quality issues that are not solely academically driven, but are driven by measures of outcome of which product fitness for purpose will be an essential element (Chapter 8). Similarly, it would be naive to think that education will be immune from the whole issue of cost-effectiveness and value for money, and so the process of contracting will allow for close scrutiny of those aspects of the colleges' services. Contracting will always operate within an environment of resource constraint and cost containment and therefore within the purchasing agenda; whoever those purchasers might be in the future, there will be issues of competing demands, prioritization and rationing to be addressed in order to support the required innovations and developments in education that will work hand in glove with developments in the health care service overall.

A successful college will be one who can get inside the business of the trust – and not just the business of today but the business of the future.

REFERENCES

Audit Commission (1991) *The Virtue of Patients: Making the best use of Ward Nursing Resources*, HMSO, London.

Butler, P. and Millar, B. (1992) No gain without pain. *Health Service Journal*, **25 June**, 10–11.

Cavanagh S. (1989) Nursing turnover: literature review and methodology critique. *Journal of Advanced Nursing*, **14**, 587–589.

Cavanagh S. (1990) Predictors of nursing staff turnover. *Journal of Advanced Nursing*, **15**, 373–380.

Conroy, M. and Stidson, M. (1988) 2001 – The black hole: an examination of labour market trends in relation to the NHS. A report from the Regional Manpower Planners Group.

Department of Health (1987) *Promoting Better Health*, HMSO, London.

Department of Health (1989a) *Caring for People*, HMSO, London.

Department of Health (1989b) *Working for Patients*, HMSO, London.

Department of Health (1989c) *Report on the Second Advisory Committee for Medical Manpower Planning*, HMSO, London.

Department of Health (1990) *Heads of Agreement, Ministerial Group on Junior Doctors' Hours*, HMSO, London.

Department of Health (1993) *Making London Better*, HMSO, London.

DHSS (Department of Health and Social Security) (1986) *Mix and Match – A Review of Nursing Skill Mix*, HMSO, London.

Heginbotham, C. (1992) Jam tomorrow. *Health Service Journal*, **5 Mar**, 24–25.

Kanter, R.M. (1989) *When Giants Learn to Dance*, Unwin, London.

King's Fund Commission on the Future of London's Acute Health Services (1992) *London Health Care 2010: Changing the Future of Service in the Capital*, Kings Fund, London.

Robinson, R. *et al.* (1992) A footholder in fundholding. *Health Service Journal*, **13 Feb**, 18–20.

Salter, B. (1991) Demand and fallacy. *Health Service Journal*, **5 December**, 19.

Stanwick, S.C. (1993) Can nurses learn to dance? Nursing and 'managed competition', in *Managing The Internal Market*, (ed. I. Tilley), Paul Chapman Publishing, London.

Tomlinson Report (1992) *Report of the Inquiry into London Health Service*, HMSO, London.

von Otter, C. (1991) The application of market principles to health care, in *Paradoxes in Competition for Health*, Nuffield Institute for Health Services Studies, University of Leeds, Leeds.

8 | Case study: incorporation and the responsive college

Bobbi Ramsammy and John Humphreys

Editors' introduction

This chapter illustrates the extent to which business practices and market awareness now inform the actions of senior education managers.

Within the context of a case study on incorporation the market is examined in relation to its implications for the structure and functioning of an education provider organization.

INTRODUCTION

The idea of a college of nursing and midwifery or of health care studies as a 'business' is a fairly new one. In this chapter consideration is given to the features of such a business that will enable it to function within the current and future health and social care delivery systems. Concepts related to marketing are explored and features of the corporate college that can effect responsiveness and the relevance to clients of education and training provision are elucidated.

These include:

1. Leadership and management;
2. Organizational structure;
3. Staff roles and responsibility, preparation, support and development;
4. Quality issues.

We will illustrate our consideration of these issues and their practical application by reference to aspects of the incorporation of Thames College of Health Care Studies into the University of Greenwich, which we successfully completed on 1 January 1993. (Other aspects of this incorporation are reported elsewhere – Whittaker *et al.*, 1994; Humphreys and Ramsammy, 1994.)

THE DEVELOPMENT OF THE MARKET

NHS reforms consequent to the White Paper *Working for Patients* (Secretaries of State, 1989) introduced to health care service and education providers the concepts of the internal market, the notion of which had been developed in theory during the 1980s (Butler, 1992). A series of working papers published by the Department of Health later on during 1989 gave further details of how the market would work (Department of Health, 1989). The main concept underlying the introduction of the internal market in respect of service provision was the separation of decisions about identifying and commissioning services to meet the needs for health care from those about the delivery of health care, the 'purchaser/provider split'. As has been explored earlier (Chapter 7), the primary concept underlying the introduction of market forces into health care education was the removal of the costs of education and training from health care service delivery pricing decisions, the so called 'level playing field'. Central to the internal market concepts were expectations of competition between providers, be they service or education, thereby increasing efficiency and reducing costs.

These concepts were new to many nurse and midwifery education providers and some influential senior educators at the time questioned their applicability (Hooper, 1990). Indeed, only the previous year the DHSS had encouraged national and regional collaboration and sharing between colleges of nursing and midwifery in the introduction of Project 2000, through the creation of demonstration districts. It might appear to some that some parts of the DHSS were not aware of what others were doing, or that the concepts of marketing were ill understood at the time by those who were leading the reforms. Be that as it may, those in senior positions within colleges were faced with identifying the 'business' that they were in and some new skills associated with planning and running a business.

Consideration of the 'mission' of the college was often not a new activity but now the situation had changed. Previously the purpose of the college had been to serve the education and training needs of one or more district health authorities (Miles, 1988). The Director of Nurse Education and staff of the college were employees of the district health authority, often managed by the Chief Nurse or Director of Personnel; thus 'Nurse education had a breadth of functions unrivalled in a Health Authority, but subordinate to all others in power and authority terms' (Rider, quoted in Miles, 1988).

In this scenario the mission of the college was determined by the strategic and operational direction of the district health authority and more often than not the objectives of service provision took precedence over those of education provision. For instance, the buildings in which nursing and midwifery education was delivered were rarely adequately maintained, as the needs of patient care areas took precedence, and whole intakes of students were regularly cut to save money in any particular financial year, often with little thought for the long-term consequences. There was therefore often little point in attempting to make separate or independent educational plans in this climate. Other issues such as the types of experiences which could be offered, shortages of staff and low numbers of trained staff on wards, outdated philosophies and approaches to care often dominated the types of course that could be run. Curriculum planning from educational principles was dominated by the need to consider the learner as worker and to provide an even flow of students through wards to meet the needs of service provision. The differing perspectives and objectives between service and education providers had in many instances during the previous decades resulted in a 'service/education' divide, often characterized by poor relations between the 'school' and the wards.

It was with this historical and cultural background that colleges of nursing and midwifery or health care studies set about identifying a 'mission' for an educational and training entity that was to provide services to a range of 'clients', i.e. mainly directly managed units (DMUs) and NHS trusts, based on an identification of their needs. In the early days of the reforms the senior staff of the DMU or trust were in a learning position themselves. In an organization in the throes of major change, many of the less senior staff were either unaware of, or actively opposed to, the reforms. The demands made on purchasers and providers was accurately predicted by Appleby *et al.* (1990) when they observed: 'Given the distinct lack of detailed prescription in the NHS reforms, the tight implementation timetable and the scope of the change, the attitudes and cultural upheavals will be particularly acute in the NHS. Health authorities, their managers, clinicians and others, face a radical change in their roles if the ideas of the reforms are to become reality'.

Many of the service providers were unsure of their future service requirements and had not begun to think of the training needs of staff. This made the position for the educators doubly difficult: an entirely different perspective and set of skills was required – those of business planning in an environment where the customers were unsure what they wanted to buy! The new skills required at that time included market analysis, market research, marketing effectiveness and contracting. Alongside this the new principals and their staff had to consider the roles of powerful 'stakeholders', e.g. the regional health authority which had responsibility for Working Paper 10 contracting. Also important in delivering the educational services was consideration of the needs of the 'consumers' (students) and the requirements of statutory and validating bodies (e.g. UKCC, ENB) and the higher education establishment. The ultimate consumer of the services of both health care delivery and health care education systems is, of course, the patient, and plans should also consider an analysis of the needs of national and local communities – all of this being provided within an environment sensitive to the resource implications of the decisions taken. So costing and pricing of services became key questions and issues surrounding the 'true' costs of education and training came even more into the spotlight. Analyses of teacher and support staff activity and effectiveness were carried out in many of the colleges. Ultimately there developed a greater awareness of public accountability and the need for financial probity. The Comptroller and Auditor General, reflecting on this period, concluded that: 'the current developments in the financing and organization of nursing education should provide a better framework for achieving value for money' (National Audit Office, 1992).

If a college was to survive and succeed in these times of major change in service delivery there was a need to develop a vision and clear sense of purpose. For the staff of the new colleges a strong corporate image and sense of belonging needed to be nurtured. Staff had to be committed to achieving the goals of the organization and of working in a creative, innovative environment.

At the same time major changes were occurring in the organization, management, structure, control and delivery aspects of nursing and midwifery education itself. Most of these changes had been triggered by the introduction of Project 2000 and the requirement that these courses be delivered at an appropriate academic level, usually Diploma of Higher Education (UKCC, 1986; ENB, 1989). For many colleges this necessitated the formation of a 'link' with an institution of higher education, and for some colleges this link provided a range of resources which were to prove helpful in achieving the massive agenda they were facing.

As a minimum the 'link' between nursing and midwifery education and higher education was for conjoint validation of courses (ENB, 1989), but many colleges took advantage of this relationship to extend provision for the students and access to the services of the higher education institution, for example teaching, library, computing, counselling etc., for the Project 2000 students (NFER, 1993). The English National Board (1989) identified a range of the benefits of such links including research, scholarship and educational development, and in particular the benefits to nursing practice were asserted: 'Such links will provide an atmosphere which encourages the questioning approach to learning in a robust acknowledgement of thinking, reflection and contemplation as ways of advancing professional knowledge as a basis for safe practice' (Akinsanya, 1990).

As working relationships developed between the staff of colleges and those of the higher education institution other benefits became obvious, for instance the benefits of flexible academic structures applied to vocational courses. Many colleges introduced diploma and degree level provision within credit accumulation and transfer schemes for student midwives and in post-registration pathways. The English National Board proposals for a higher award (ENB, 1991) and the UKCC consultation papers on post-registration education for professional practice (UKCC, 1990), both advocated development of unitized educational programmes within a credit accumulation and transfer scheme. Those higher education establishments which were able to offer these opportunities were sought out by a range of colleges of nursing and midwifery and other educational and professional bodies (Chapters 3 and 4). The colleges of nursing and midwifery or of health care studies that were fortunate enough to have established close working relationships with leaders in the field of credit and accreditation found themselves in the position of being market leaders themselves as educational opportunities mushroomed.

At almost the same time as these developments were taking place questions were being asked about the future management of the colleges. As continued management within NHS structures was no longer appropriate nor possible (Department of Health, 1991) the viable alternative for many colleges was seen to be incorporation into the higher education institution, often preceded or accompanied by amalgamation of two or more schools or colleges into one (Booth, 1992). These amalgamations and incorporations or mergers, while challenging the skills of educational leaders in the management of major organizational change and causing anxiety and stress amongst staff delivering the educational services, gave opportunities to consider how a range of aspects in the organization, management and running of the new corporate college/faculty might contribute to increased effectiveness in responding to the needs of customers. These aspects would include:

1. organizational structures and the roles and responsibilities of staff to enhance customer relations and market effectiveness;
2. staff development programmes to address preparation of staff for the changes, for the different perspective that consideration of internal and external markets and customer relations requires and the development of an organizational culture which enhances effectiveness;
3. quality management concepts and their application to the delivery of educational services;
4. design of services to maintain market responsiveness and share.

ORGANIZATIONAL STRUCTURES AND MARKET EFFECTIVENESS

Many of the management 'gurus' of the 1980s and 1990s have considered the effects of various organizational structures on the effectiveness of businesses and services. On the whole management theorists have agreed that bureaucratic structures characterized by hierarchy of authority, with many layers of middle managers and long chains of command, lengthy decision making, cumbersome communication processes and standardized work processes are not flexible enough to respond appropriately to customers' needs. Most district health authorities and their schools of nursing in the early 1980s would have exhibited the characteristics associated with bureaucratic organizational structures. Miles (1988) described a typical structure of a school of nursing and highlighted some of the problems of liaison and accountability that notions of hierarchy caused.

These problems were occurring at a time when most schools of nursing and midwifery were relatively small by today's standards. Many were serving the educational needs of only one or two district health authorities and had fairly limited, largely non-accredited post-basic and continuing education provision. As the size and complexity of schools increased during the latter years of the 1980s, many schools/colleges instituted matrix or modified matrix structures in an attempt to overcome these problems. Whatever the structure the overriding message is that to be effective there is the need to 'get close to the customer, find out what they want, and give it to them'.

Peters and Waterman (1982) report that their research revealed excellent companies to be: 'close to their customers and ... focused on service, quality, listening to their users and developing niche markets'. They went on to describe the characteristics of the 'structure of the 80s' with three pillars:

1. **stability** – to respond to the need for efficiency in the basics;
2. **entrepreneurship** – to respond to the need for innovation;
3. **'habit breaking'** – to respond to the need to avoid calcification.

Later in the decade Peters (1987) described a flat structure, with all functional barriers broken, in which self-managed teams find ways to connect responsively to local customers. New attitudes of total customer responsiveness involving closer linkages with and listening to customers were recommended. Customer information systems at both formal and informal levels are seen to be as important as, if not more important than, management information systems.

More recently Hooper (1990) recommended that a central prerequisite for success in the inevitable process of change is the need to reorganize to facilitate integration and to create departments responsive to new activities, removing unnecessary layers of management.

In managing the merger of Thames College of Health Care Studies with the University of Greenwich we established a working group to decide on the structure most likely to reflect the health care needs of our DMU and Trust clients, the educational needs of our 'consumers' (the students on a wide variety of educational programmes), while at the same time being able to work effectively within the university. The need to keep a close focus on health rather than purely higher education issues when managing incorporation is reflected in the National Audit Office's advice to consider the following issues as important for health authorities planning to transfer their college to higher education:

1. maintenance of the health service input into nursing education;
2. ability to influence student recruitment policies;
3. determination of quality and performance standards;
4. reporting arrangements (National Audit Office, 1992).

The academic organization and committee structure of the university provided a framework for the delivery of courses, based on schools as the major functional unit. Schools provide an academic base for all staff, students and courses. Convenient groupings of related schools into faculties allows the coordination of resourcing and developments, and the operation of quality control mechanisms.

Each school is responsible for delivery of 'courses' within the university's credit framework. In fact, as we shall see later, there was rapid growth during this period of faculty-wide undergraduate and postgraduate credit schemes and a proliferation of pathways and units within the schemes, as well as major developments across faculties. Thus notions of free-standing self-contained courses soon became defunct.

In the university many schools also grouped staff into academic disciplines or areas of study called divisions, with the purpose of encouraging subject development, research, consultancy and scholarly work. The position of Head of Division is seen as complementary to that of Course Director, taking on responsibility for subject leadership together with administrative responsibilities for academic staff within the division. It was this concept that we decided would be useful for the College of Health Care Studies/Faculty of Health designate (hereafter referred to as the Faculty of Health) to apply in 'getting close to the customer'.

Three aspects of school structure and function will now be considered in more detail.

Clinical directorate-focused divisions

The mission of the faculty is to: 'develop as a centre of excellence providing high quality, cost effective, flexible and contemporary education and training in health and social care in response to identified needs, and contributing actively to research and development' (Faculty of Health, 1993).

In order to ensure the provision of high-quality, cost-effective, flexible and contemporary education and training in response to identified needs we decided that it was essential for members of senior staff in the faculty to be given responsibilities for ensuring that day-to-day communications were effected with health service clinicians and managers. These staff would need to have an intimate knowledge of the service provider's business, be credible at an executive level and have time to liaise at a range of levels and on a variety of issues with their service counterparts. For these reasons we considered that they should not also have responsibility for course delivery or for managing the experience of students. We therefore devised a structure which separated these two functions (Figure 8.1).

Responsibility for course/pathway delivery was divided between two schools, Pre-Registration and Post-Registration – which later were renamed 'Initial Professional and Vocational Health Studies' and 'Advanced Professional Health Studies'. Each school also provided a 'home' for four clinically focused divisions and one functional centre. The divisions and centres provide a cross-faculty service to all courses, thus an internal market exists within the faculty.

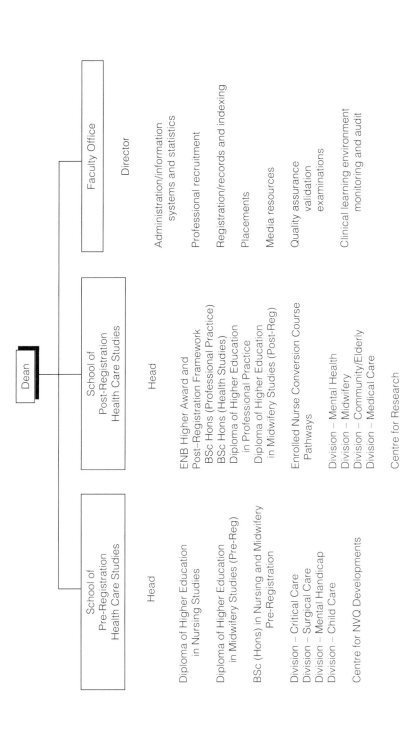

Figure 8.1 Structure of the Faculty of Health at the time of incorporation into the University of Greenwich. Each school contains programmes of study and distinct clinically focused divisions.

Divisional staff have a specific external focus with our main clients, i.e. those directly managed units and NHS trusts for whom the regional health authority commission education and training. Some divisions also liaise with other clients such as the private, voluntary and independent sectors. By participating with these service providers in activities such as training needs analysis and clinical audit (with particular emphasis on clinical learning environment issues) senior staff in the faculty can gather vital marketing information to ensure that the educational services provided are relevant to their clients. Training needs analysis gives them an opportunity to proactively influence contracting through knowledge of the service provider's 'business' and assisting in consideration of issues such as skill mix and service delivery patterns. They are also able to continuously provide feedback on quality issues through the information provided by clinical learning environment audit. Collaborative research between educationalists and service providers can also serve to enhance patient care and highlight educational needs for clients and carers. While carrying out these activities they are also able to act as intelligence gatherers regarding service developments and changes in policies as well as being able to feed back to the faculty managers and course directors any issues regarding current delivery of educational provision. They provide a vital communication channel between the faculty and service providers.

As well as the external focus detailed above, divisions also have a major responsibility in the faculty for coordinating the work of the teachers within their specialty area and ensuring that high quality teaching is provided for 'courses'. This role is enacted by the heads of division and their deputies acting as subject leaders responsible for the development of the subject, its delivery and monitoring. Thus they have to be aware of the demands of both the internal and external markets. Significantly in developing divisions as clinically focused, we rejected the alternate possibility that they should be academically derived (biology, social science etc.).

Management of the student experience

In this structure, scheme, course and pathway leaders are freed from the need to coordinate and manage the processes detailed above to concentrate on ensuring the provision of high quality experiences to the other major players in the arena – the 'consumers', i.e. the students. Students are often influential in determining the views and perceptions of health care service managers regarding the services being provided by the faculty, either directly through feedback to the managers about the quality of the educational provision or indirectly through their performance in clinical areas. Current students are also an important factor in recruiting new students. Word of mouth has been identified as the single most important factor in determining choice of training school (Miles, 1981). Having undertaken one course within the faculty they may also provide for a significant aspect of repeat business, particularly if the experience has been positive.

Therefore the role of the course managers in an environment that is responsive to students needs is an extremely important one. This does not mean that course managers have no role in customer relations, marketing and market research but that this is not their primary focus.

Centres for development of specific aspects of the faculty's work

The final components of the structure which we devised are the two centres, one for NVQ developments, and one for health research and ethics. These centres were designed to provide an internal and external focus for areas of work within their remit. The centre for NVQ development, as well as running City and Guilds accredited courses for health and social care support workers, provides preparation courses for assessors and internal verifiers for assessment of competence. Staff of the centre are also involved in local and international developments in relation to NVQs and latterly GNVQs. Although not necessarily higher education, these activities are considered a very important part of the faculty provision. By offering such facilities in addition to other more mainstream activities, the faculty is in a position to offer a relatively full service to client trusts ranging from Health Care Assistant through to research and consultancy.

The Health Research and Ethics Centre was set up to ensure development in the faculty in an area of work which was relatively new to us, but which rapidly assumed major importance, particularly following incorporation. The centre provides a focus for subject specialist development and delivery as well as for collaborative research with clinical areas and other faculties. Work in the centre follows three main themes, community and primary health care, analysis of innovations and developments in health care delivery programmes and evaluation of health care education delivery.

Both centres also provide advice to other staff of the faculty on issues related to their work.

ROLES AND RESPONSIBILITIES OF ACADEMIC STAFF

When devising this structure managers of the college/faculty were aware of the danger of course managers becoming divorced from their colleagues in divisions and losing touch with clinical developments. In order to overcome potential problems in this area all faculty managers and scheme/pathway/course leaders are 'affiliated' to an appropriate division. Affiliated staff are expected to carry out the same roles and responsibilities as any other member of staff of a division but due regard is taken of the demands of their other roles and responsibilities. The roles and responsibilities of all academic staff were clearly defined to minimize confusion, to enhance coordination of the various activities in which we were involved and to ensure responsibility and accountability for separate aspects of our functions. These roles are now explored in greater detail as is the contribution of each individual in the corporate responsive college/faculty to its success.

Clarity in the understanding of roles is highlighted by Dixon (1993) as an often neglected area in the health service. She identified organization structure as the explicit and shared understandings of roles, the contribution of these roles in an organization and relationships in terms of authority and accountability. She went on to point out that it has become unfashionable to focus on structure and that some of the ills besetting the private and public sectors might be attributed to overfocusing on the 'warm and cuddly' approaches to management stressing interpersonal relations and teamwork. She concludes: 'It is not an exaggeration to suggest that much of the current malaise and inefficiency in the private and public sectors arises from an unwillingness to clarify who is accountable for what and to whom'.

Within the college we subscribed to the importance of role clarification within the overall structure; however, as will be examined in more detail later, this did not entirely overcome problems associated with role confusion. As previously mentioned all academic staff were expected to fulfil four primary responsibilities or functions, no matter what their individual role or position within the faculty. These four responsibilities are:

1. teaching in a nursing or midwifery specialist area;
2. teaching in an academic discipline or study area one of the subjects underpinning and applied to the study of nursing or midwifery;
3. acting as personal tutor to a number of students;
4. fulfilling a clinical liaison role within specified clinical areas.

In addition to these four core responsibilities academic staff are expected to undertake a range of additional responsibilities as well as fulfilling requirements for research and scholarly activity (albeit linked with their clinical and/or academic specialist area).

When incorporation occurred and all academic staff of the College of Health Care Studies took up university conditions of employment, it was agreed that staff of the Faculty of Health would, in common with academic staff in other disciplines, normally complete up to 550 hours of direct contact with students per year. It was decided that these hours would be used to fulfil the first three of the core responsibilities, and that no teacher would be expected to undertake these activities for more than 38 weeks of the year, i.e. a teacher would spend up to 14.5 hours a week in direct contact with students. Alongside this, faculty managers set out to ensure that teachers were able to assist the service staff in developing clinical environments conducive to the learning needs of all staff in the area as well as influencing the care given to patients/clients. We introduced a policy which 'contracted' teachers to spend on average 7.5 hours per week, 45 weeks of the year, in clinical liaison activity, with clearly defined responsibilities to carry out in the clinical area.

In order to coordinate this range of very complex relationships, both within the faculty and with our clients, and to ensure that we were able to comply with university requirements, we set up a formal committee structure. Most of our committees serve to provide for smooth internal operations, formal communications, coordination of resources, quality assurance, monitoring and feedback. One important committee, though, has a specific external focus, the Faculty Advisory Committee. Its terms of reference are: a) to maintain effective consultative mechanisms on which to base the direction of curriculum development and other services; b) to facilitate contract negotiations; and c) to generally inform the faculty's strategic and operational planning. The Committee comprises members from local health service purchasers and providers, the regional health authority, family health services authorities, GP fundholders, local secondary schools, the English National Board, private, voluntary and independent sectors and community health councils. The committee meets twice a year, chaired by the Dean of Faculty and provides a valuable source of information about current and future work. Although important in strategic terms, this committee merely sits at the top of a whole college structure designed to facilitate an intimate and widespread understanding of trust needs.

STAFF PREPARATION AND DEVELOPMENT

The structures described were implemented late in 1992 at the same time as changes were occurring in the NHS generally and in London specifically. In higher education the binary division had been removed and our higher education partner became a university (it had formally been Thames Polytechnic). Changes were also happening in health and social care working practices; for example, reductions in junior doctors' hours and the consequent changes in the scope of professional practice for nurses; the introduction of community care reforms with the shift of responsibility for needs assessment from health services to social services. All these factors made very great demands on the staff of the college, particularly with regard to the development of different working practices. At the same time as introducing this new structure the college was almost ready for incorporation into the university and staff were concerned about pay and conditions of service. Many of the new roles they were to undertake involved a move of base, and they were also being introduced to a new culture, that of higher education. Every effort had been made to prepare them for the changes (Humphreys and Ramsammy, 1994; Whittaker et al., 1994) through a variety of activities, e.g.: distribution of information about the university; large-scale staff meetings and workshops; an incorporation newsletter; bookable 'one-to-one' interviews with senior managers; presentations about the university; and 'pairing' staff as they were appointed to posts in the new structure with 'partners' in the university. A further series of meetings was held just before the new structure was implemented specifically targeted on heads of division and 'course' managers.

Despite these efforts the first few months after implementation were extremely difficult for all staff. It appeared that anything that could go wrong did go wrong! There were tensions between the divisions and the courses, systems of work broke down, information flow between colleagues was not good and signs of conflict abounded. This despite very thorough preparation.

INCORPORATION AS PROJECT MANAGEMENT

The detailed and focused work surrounding incorporation of the College of Health Care Studies into the University of Greenwich began in earnest in February 1992. Prior to that date the Board of Management of the college had commissioned a working group to carry out an options appraisal on the future status, organization and management of the college. This group produced an interim report in July 1991 and a final report in November 1991. The interim report recommended that the college should become a faculty: 'subject to satisfactory outcomes to further work on:

- the structure, organization and management of the Faculty;
- personnel arrangements for staff transferring into the Faculty;
- financial arrangements between South East Thames Regional Health Authority, Bexley, Dartford and Gravesham and Greenwich Health Authorities and the Polytechnic;
- transfer of responsibility for capital and other assets currently used by the College from the Districts to the Polytechnic' (Final Report of the Working Group, November 1991).

The strategies used to tackle these aspects of the incorporation project illustrate some of the ways in which leadership and management can contribute to success in achieving the necessary changes, and demonstrate how some of the issues surrounding the integration of colleges of health into higher education can be resolved.

The working group considered that a steering group should be set up to coordinate and manage the implementation of the above recommendations. In order to ensure that agreed work was carried out and that action could be taken speedily without the need to constantly refer back to 'higher authorities' it was decided that the membership be drawn from executive managers of the three district health authorities, the polytechnic and the college. The steering group was chaired by the regional officer with delegated responsibility for non-nursing Working Paper 10 funding; this facilitated access to regional services and personnel at appropriate times and provided a neutral/objective overview to the whole process. As will be described later other members were coopted to the steering group as and when necessary.

The timescales set for the steering group to achieve its task were very tight, i.e. 7 months.

The principles adopted by the steering group in achieving its goals were:

1. **to ensure action**, i.e. that at the end of every meeting members were clear as to what they were expected to achieve;
2. **to maintain open communication with staff at all times** through the mechanisms previously described;
3. **to protect the position of all staff** so that no one should find her/himself financially disadvantaged by the incorporation;
4. **to ensure that neither the health authorities nor the university should take commercial gain from the incorporation**.

Various mechanisms were put into place to assist this: for instance, the member of staff of the university who had been most closely involved with the college since its inception was appointed Honorary Vice-Principal. This was primarily seen as important in helping to finalize the faculty management structure, agreeing staff appointments and continuing communications and staff development strategies. In the event the person who fulfilled this role participated fully in all aspects of the incorporation work and proved a valuable resource on a wide range of issues. The college's Principal was charged with the day-to-day responsibility for ensuring that the incorporation proceeded smoothly. To facilitate this a member of the senior management team of the college was appointed as full-time Project Officer, assisted by a full-time temporary secretary.

In addition, an Incorporation Project Team was formed, the members of which were: the college Principal, the Honorary Vice-Principal, the Project Officer, personnel officers of the college and the polytechnic, the chair of the staff representative group (the Incorporation Advisory Group), the member of the senior management team of the college who had specific responsibility for staff development and two project researchers who investigated aspects of the incorporation.

Finally an Incorporation Advisory Group (IAG) was set up to enable all staff to have speedy feedback from the steering group (the chair of the IAG was coopted as a full member of the steering group), and to ensure that any concerns of staff were answered and, if possible, quickly resolved. In addition 'incorporation' and progress towards it became a standing agenda item on every formal meeting within the college for the duration of the project.

The steering group met first in February 1992 and made an interim report to the health authorities in May/June advising that the original date for incorporation, i.e. September, could not be met due to lack of clarity about conditions of staff transfer. The final report of the steering group was made in October/November to the three health authorities and to the university Court of Governors who all agreed to the recommendations in the report. These recommendations concluded that Thames College of Health Care Studies should be incorporated into the University of Greenwich as the Faculty of Health on or before 1 January 1993.

In making this recommendation the steering group kept uppermost in their considerations the need to ensure that the faculty is able to: a) respond speedily, flexibly and efficiently to health care service providers' education and training needs; b) maintain close working relationships with service providers; c) enhance the quality of education and training; and d) ensure continuity of delivery through incorporation.

With regard to personnel issues the steering group considered and rejected the possibility of long term secondment of staff from the NHS and of staff remaining members of the NHS pension scheme and enjoying Whitley Council terms and conditions of service while in the employ of the university. The recommendation made was that all staff be offered University of Greenwich contracts of employment on university terms and conditions of service.

The university managers had indicated that they were prepared to offer salaries and terms and conditions that were no less favourable than those currently enjoyed. The steering group had examined the similarities and differences between the two pension schemes and were satisfied that staff would not be disadvantaged. Staff who transferred to university employment were able to transfer their accrued pension rights in full to the university scheme. Staff who enjoyed Mental Health Officer status had an enhanced service credit to reflect the higher accrual rate of their pension benefits in the NHS scheme. Alternatively, staff were able to choose to have their pension rights preserved with full inflation-proofing until retirement age. The regional health authority indicated willingness to make up any differences in pension transfer on an individual basis, either by buying additional years or by taking out pension plans.

The university indicated preparedness to recognize individual staff members' length of service for the purpose of sick or maternity leave, redundancy or other benefits. The steering group was confident that no member of the College's staff would be disadvantaged financially or in employment terms by these arrangements.

Staff were kept informed and up to date about incorporation issues and had opportunities to express their worries and concerns to the college's managers and to the steering group. Professional organizations and trade union representatives were also regularly consulted regarding proposals and offered constructive advice and information about similar incorporation proposals across the country.

We ourselves (Humphreys and Ramsammy, 1994) have taken the view that in the new competitive climate of health care education 'surviving incorporation' is:

> not simply about staff contracts, buildings, finance and academic structures. It is as much as anything about creating a group of people with the capacity to thrive in a difficult and competitive market. Just as colleges need to be most effective in order to maintain their business, they are being subjected to the stresses and anxieties of incorporation. In these circumstances, the quality of the incorporation may have long-term significance. It is quite possible that the resilience of some colleges will be severely challenged by the twin tests of incorporation and competition.

LEADERSHIP AND MANAGEMENT IN THE CORPORATE COLLEGE

We have already identified that an organizational climate or culture which fosters innovation and creativity in response to identified needs should be developed through appropriate leadership techniques and staff development programmes. Hooper (1990) identifies that: 'a successful School of Nursing and Midwifery will have a culture through which staff learn to adapt to, and cope with, external pressure'. Webster (1990) argues that an organization's ability to respond to change is dependent upon the prevailing culture within it, Edwards (1993) adds that colleges of nursing will need to develop: 'a progressive organizational culture that is decentralized, flexible, goal-directed and participative, where individuals are seen as partners working towards a common objective'.

Leadership which enables this type of culture to develop and flourish has been referred to as 'transformational'. One of the most influential and successful leaders of nursing education in this period advocates sound two-way communication, action plans to achieve goals and regular 'time out' to share problems and issues as ways of managing change during the implementation of one of the pilot Project 2000 courses (Hooper, 1990). What seems to be important in her account of the dynamic and innovative college that she led was a climate and culture which could sustain effort in an ever-changing environment.

It has been suggested that the current climate of change makes different demands from previously on those in leadership and management roles, and that failure to recognize these needs and demands can have catastrophic effects on individuals and organizations.

> The adaptive corporation needs a new kind of leadership. It needs 'managers of adaptation' equipped with a whole new set of non-linear skills. Above all the adaptive manager today must be willing to think beyond the thinkable – to reconceptualize products, procedures, programmes, and purposes before crisis makes drastic change inescapable.
>
> Warned of impending upheaval, most managers still pursue business as usual. Yet business as usual is dangerous in an environment that has become permanently convulsive. (Toffler, 1985)

In our college, which was undertaking restructuring prior to incorporation, the senior management team set out to try as far as possible to equip ourselves and our staff to meet the challenges and changes before us as positively as possible. On the one hand it was necessary to ensure throughout the changes that we did pursue 'business' as usual, i.e. we had to continue to deliver our contracted work. There was a tendency to resist developing new initiatives during this time, particularly from some of the less experienced staff or those who had not fully appreciated the new situation. However those in more senior management positions recognized that we could not wait a year to 18 months to address some of the issues confronting us. We compromised by agreeing that only the most pressing developments would go on during this period.

Managing the changes detailed above stretched the skills and abilities of the college's senior management team to an unprecedented degree. As this college was amongst the first to make the transition there was little guidance from the Department of Health or from the statutory bodies. The English National Board has now produced a good practice guide for integrating nursing and midwifery education into higher education (ENB, 1993), which should prove helpful to those college principals and their senior management teams who are at the beginning of this process. Nevertheless leaders and managers will still have to work through these issues and others and tackle problems post-incorporation for which many are ill equipped through lack of targeted development. In the authors' opinion the future preparation of those who lead and manage colleges or faculties of nursing and midwifery or health care studies or their equivalent needs careful consideration.

It is the authors' contention that current leaders within the nursing profession need to review the pros and cons of the options facing nursing/midwifery/health care education management in the future, take a view as to which is the most appropriate and ensure that there are sufficient appropriately prepared people to lead and manage nursing and midwifery education for that future. There is at present a gap in research studies on the organization and management of nursing and midwifery education within the United Kingdom which should be rectified as soon as possible. Gough (1992) considers the current changes in nurse education in the wider context of organizational and managerial change, technological style and socio-institutional arrangements and also reflects on the limited literature and paucity of public debate within the profession on the issues.

The importance of the leadership and management role of the principals/deans of colleges or faculties of nursing and midwifery education during a time of major change should not be underestimated. There is some evidence to suggest that, in the past, preparation for this role has been somewhat haphazard. In England, in 1983, the National Staff Committee for Nurses and Midwives, concerned at the lack of suitable candidates for Director of Nurse Education (DNE) posts set up a project designed to prepare prospective DNEs for their role. More recently the English National Board has recognized the importance of staff development for the principals of colleges of nursing and midwifery and has commissioned a series of workshops and standing conferences. Goldenberg (1990) describes similar problems with nursing education leadership in Canada, emphasizing that there is an 'educational crisis' in both the preparation for the role and the number of vacant positions. Similarly the lack of leadership or management or both within universities in several countries is commented upon by Daniel (1988), who suggests that institutional researchers can help to improve leadership in higher education.

Scott and Jaffe (1989) indicate the magnitude of the changes required for today's leaders and managers:

In the past, the definition of management competence rested on specific management planning, scheduling, and controlling techniques. Today, competence is based more on attitudes, approaches, philosophies, values and the ability to create improvements in health, innovation, and productivity. A manager today is playing a different game, and must manage in a different way. He or she must be a change manager, or, better a change leader. Change leadership is not a skill reserved for top management. As organizations struggle to respond to the pressures of competition, you and your work team have to learn to move quickly in order to attain higher standards and increased productivity.

Miles *et al.* (1988) explore how knowledge of theory relating to organizational climate, culture and health can inform educational leaders. In an analysis of culture Miles and Snow (1978) explored four typologies related to business.

1. The first of these typologies, **defenders**, serve narrow, stable market segments and tend to grow by increasing their shares within their target markets. They ignore developments outside their target markets and in companies exhibiting 'defender' traits there is very little development of new products or new markets. Structures in these organizations are simple and decision-making is centralized.
2. By contrast, the second typology, **prospectors**, serve broadly defined dynamic markets and grow by generating new products and identifying new markets. They are continually identifying unsatisfied consumer needs and creating products to satisfy those needs. In these organizations there is a continuing developing capacity to monitor a wide range of environmental conditions, trends and events. Decision-making is decentralized and structures are complex.
3. **Analysers**, the third typology, have characteristics of both defenders and prospectors and serve a mixture of stable and changing markets. On measures of innovation they occupy the middle ground; they make fewer and slower product or market changes and are less committed to stability and efficiency than defenders. In order to move quickly towards a new product or market that has gained a 'degree of acceptance' they use extensive market surveillance mechanisms. Structures in these organizations are a combination of simple and complex and decision-making is moderately centralized.
4. The fourth typology, **reactors**, lack a clearly defined strategic focus and frequently change their business definition and scope.

One would imagine that colleges of nursing and midwifery or of health care studies exhibiting characteristics of defenders or reactors in today's climate would not last long. They would need to change to an analyser or prospector mode in order to survive. Leaders and managers of these organizations must ensure that the required changes take place or risk the inevitable consequences. It seems to us that one of the key areas of the work of the college or faculty that the leader should focus on, to address the changes necessary, is that of quality.

QUALITY IN A CORPORATE PARADIGM

The concept of quality is one for which it is difficult to agree a universally acceptable definition. Attree (1993) has analysed the concept and identifies several interpretations of quality: excellence; ideal; fitness for purpose and conformance to standards; meeting the customer's requirements; satisfying need; and customer value.

In a responsive college it is important to consider definitions of quality and to identify which approach is being taken so that all staff are working towards common goals with shared values. In the new Faculty of Health we decided that our major approach to quality should be in terms of meeting the customers' requirements and providing customer value.

The concept of customer value has, according to Attree, become associated with a 'marketplace economic philosophy', i.e. if customers do not perceive a product or service as good value then they will take their custom elsewhere. When the NHS reforms came into place and Working Paper 10 became a reality it seemed to us that the logical consequence of these changes was that a college could 'go out of business' if contracts were not placed with it. Unlike some of our neighbouring colleges we had few other 'quality' attributes to commend us: we were not part of a 'prestigious' London teaching hospital; there was no tradition of research or of academic or scholarly work; we did not offer education and training to a wide range of health service personnel. We did, however, have reasonably close and good relationships with our primary purchasers and we set out to capitalize on these. It was decided that we should adopt a 'fitness for purpose', framework to enable us to measure how we were achieving our goals.

The English National Board defines 'fitness for purpose' as 'judging how well an institution or course/programme is performing against its stated objectives' (ENB, 1993a). As has been argued earlier such stated objectives should reflect the needs of the clients and consumers and in the responsive faculty/college the clients and consumers should have a voice in judging how well the institution and course/programme is performing. This is not to say that the clients' view of quality is the only one to be taken into account; there are other groups who should and do have a legitimate view on the quality of an educational organization and its 'products'. These include regional Working Paper 10 'commissioners', the English National Board and the higher education establishment which conjointly validate programmes, other accrediting or validating organizations, the Higher Education Funding Council for England and the staff of the institution. Each of these individuals or groups will have their own perspective of how well an institution is doing, each may draw on different evidence from which to make judgements, and the decisions made about the effectiveness of the institution or its 'products' might differ between individuals or groups.

It is almost inevitable therefore that issues surrounding a definition of quality which focuses on 'fitness for purpose' will pose tensions for educationists in health care settings. Humphreys (1993), in an analysis of these tensions, writes:

Through all such changes of approach and attitude, a challenge for colleges will be to maintain intellectual and professional demand on students and the rigour of assessment necessary to maintain the general standard of programmes and the consequent integrity of the awards. Working for clients is not simply about complying with their wishes. Despite the rate of change, most clients and colleges will continue to work together with a degree of stability (losses and gains of business will in most cases be incremental rather than catastrophic – not least because of the length of programmes). In this context, colleges will need to establish the type of relationship where creative solutions to difficult problems emerge. Apparent tensions between costs and standards, local focus and national credibility etc. will need to be solved with both rigour and imagination.

Fitness for purpose, in our view, should also focus on the processes of education and the practitioners who have been exposed to these processes. Those who work in a responsive educational environment need to continually reflect on their own practices. To facilitate such reflection, we established a working group which has first identified some fairly universally accepted elements of quality in order to analyse and improve the quality of our services. These elements are: efficiency, effectiveness, appropriateness, accessibility and acceptability.

During the year the managers of the college had received a small sum of money from the regional health authority to investigate ways in which we might prepare ourselves for incorporation and develop our business. It was agreed that we should spend this money by focusing on three areas of the work of the faculty that we felt would enable us to make a preliminary survey of these five elements. These areas of work were finance, performance indicators and business planning. College managers had previously undertaken an analysis of the organization using a variety of tools. We had found that internal surveys were very time consuming and felt that they were not always perceived positively by staff; we also considered that we would benefit from some external views of our organization at what was a crucial point in our development. Consequently we engaged consultants to undertake preliminary analysis in the three aspects of this work.

With regard to the efficiency of the faculty we decided to examine how we used the resources at our disposal, e.g. financial, human, space; effectiveness was investigated through an analysis of the perceptions of our clients and consumers as well as the staff of the institution. While carrying out this investigation we included questions about appropriateness, accessibility and acceptability of our services.

Questionnaires were sent to all wards and departments and we carried out interviews with the managers of local trusts and directly managed units and with representatives of the student body on all of the courses that we run. The questionnaires and interviews included questions related to each of our categories. Staff were

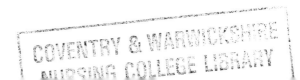

also surveyed in an effort to gain as wide as possible view of our services. While carrying out the survey we incorporated market research questions so that our future services could be planned in response to needs identified through this process. The findings of this survey indicated that, while the majority of our traditional work, i.e. teaching and assessment and closely related activities such as course planning and student support, were rated as high-quality, our ability to deal reactively and proactively with the needs of clients was still ill understood and therefore not well demonstrated by the majority of our staff. At the end of the first six months of work the quality working group recommended that we:

1. ensured that key faculty staff at all levels were identified and given specific responsibility for providing focused, timely and accurate information to service managers and clinical areas;

2. ensured that key staff who had responsibility for communication with colleagues throughout the faculty fulfilled this important part of their role;

3. ensured that existing services were maintained and improved and that planning for future courses and pathways was effected reflecting identified needs;

4. reviewed all course/pathways/units in the light of identified purchasing factors;

5. explored more flexible approaches to course delivery with respect to time and location;

6. undertook further research to match teaching and learning methods employed with student enjoyment and course/unit outcomes;

7. dealt urgently with areas of concern relating to the Diploma in Higher Education (Nursing Studies) – e.g. placements, role of the practice facilitators) – and evaluated the course's ability to deliver practitioners to meet service needs;

8. identified ways in which student facilities and resources should be improved, particularly relating to common rooms and numbers of books available;

9. devised and implemented a strategy for ensuring that all faculty staff were committed to the delivery of a high-quality service;

10. identified a senior member of staff with specific responsibility for the coordination and monitoring of matters relating to quality.

In the early summer of 1993, five months after becoming a faculty, these recommendations were agreed and the second stage of work began.

So with these matters amongst our priorities, we face an uncertain future for health care education. However some aspects of our situation now seem stable. We are part of a corporate organization (a university) offering services to other such organizations (NHS trusts). For as long as the NHS is in a state of change, so our market will be volatile and difficult to predict. In such an environment, our rate of change and speed of response will be crucial. We intend to stay in the game.

REFERENCES

Akinsanya, J. (1990) Nursing links with higher education: a prescription for change in the 21st century. *Journal of Advanced Nursing*, **15**, 744–754.

Appleby, J., Robinson, R., Ranade, W. *et al.* (1990) The use of markets in the Health Service: the NHS reforms and managed competition. *Public Money and Management*, **Winter**, 27–33.

Attree, M. (1993) An analysis of the concept 'quality' as it relates to contemporary nursing care. *International Journal of Nursing Studies*, **30**(4), 355–369.

Booth, R.A. Working for Patients: further implications for nurse education. *Nurse Education Today* **12**, 243–251.

Butler, J. (1992) *Patients, Policies and Politics. Before and After Working for Patients*, Open University Press, Milton Keynes.

Daniel, J.S. (1988) Promoting quality through leadership. Paper presented at the Association for Institutional Research Annual Conference.

Department of Health (1989) NHS Review Working Papers. (1) *Self-Governing Hospitals*. (2) *Funding and Contracts for Health Services*. (3) *Practice Budgets for General Medical Practitioners*. (4) *Indicative Prescribing Budgets for General Medical Practitioners*. (5) *Capital Charges*. (6) *Medical Audit*. (7) *NHS Consultants: Appointments, Contracts and Distinction Awards*. (8) *Implications for Family Practitioner Committees*. (9) *Capital Charges: Funding Issues* (10) *Education and Training*. HMSO, London.

Department of Health (1991) *National Health Service 'Colleges of Health' Working Party*, National Audit Office, HMSO, London.

Dixon, M. (1993) Board games. *Health Service Journal*, **29 July**, 22–23.

English National Board for Nursing, Midwifery and Health Visiting (1989) *Managing Change in Nursing Education, Pack 2*, ENB, London.

English National Board for Nursing, Midwifery and Health Visiting (1991) *Framework for Continuing Professional Education for Nurses, Midwives and Health Visitors and Higher Award*, ENB, London.

English National Board for Nursing, Midwifery and Health Visiting (1993a) *Guidelines for Educational Audit*, ENB, London.

English National Board for Nursing, Midwifery and Health Visiting (1993b) *Integrating Nursing and Midwifery Education into Higher Education*, ENB, London.

Faculty of Health (1993) University of Greenwich Mission Statement. Interim Policy Paper. Unpublished document, University of Greenwich, London.

Goldenberg, D. (1990) Nursing education leadership: effect of situational and constraint variables of leadership style. *Journal of Advanced Nursing*, **15**, 1326–1334.

Gough, P. (1992) Nurse education in the post-Fordist era. *Nurse Education Today*, **12**, 88–93.

Hooper, J. (1990) Nurse education Initiatives – making Project 2000 a reality. *Nurse Education Today*, **10**, 380–397.

Humphreys, J. (1993) The marketing gap in health care education. *Nurse Education Today*, **13**, 202–209.

Humphreys, J. and Ramsammy, R. (1994) Creating the market for health care education: an approach to college incorporation. *British Journal of Nursing*, (in press).

Miles, R.J. *et al.* (1988) *Management in Nurse Education*, Costello, Kent.

Miles, R.J. (1981) Selection for survival. A case study of selection, drop-out and wastage on an SRN training course in the West Roding District School of Nursing. University of London. MA Dissertation.

Miles, R.J. and Snow, C.C. (1978) *Organisational Strategy, Structure and Process*, McGraw-Hill, New York.

National Audit Office (1992) *Nursing Education: Implementation of Project 2000 in England*, Report by the Comptroller and Auditor General, HMSO, London.

NFER (1993) *National Evaluation of Demonstration Schemes in Pre-registration Nurse Education (Project 2000)*, HMSO, London.

Peters, T.J. (1987) *Thriving on Chaos*, Macmillan, London.

Peters, T.J. and Waterman, R.H. (1982) *In Search Of Excellence*, Harper & Row, New York.

Scott, C.D. and Jaffe, D.T. (1989) *Managing Organizational Change*, Crisp Publications, London.

Secretaries of State for Health, Wales, Northern Ireland and Scotland (1989) *Working for Patients*, Cmnd 555. HMSO, London.

Toffler, A. (1985) *The Adaptive Corporation*, Pan, London.

United Kingdom Central Council for Nursing, Midwifery and Health Visiting (1986) *Project 2000: A New Preparation for Practice*, UKCC, London.

United Kingdom Central Council for Nursing, Midwifery and Health Visiting (1990) *The Report of the Post-registration Education and Practice Project*, UKCC, London.

Webster, R. (1990) The importance of marketing in nurse education. *Nurse Education Today*, **10**, 140–144.

Whittaker, C., Dickinson, H., Humphreys, J. and Ramsammy, R. (1994) An evaluation of communication strategies during the process of incorporating a college of health care studies into a University. *Journal of Advanced Nursing Practice*, **19**, 653–658.

New models in a corporate paradigm

9

John Humphreys

Editors' introduction

This chapter returns to the paradigmatic issues raised explicitly in Chapters 1 and 2 and evidenced in the case studies and other earlier chapters.

Basic tensions between professional and 'corporate' priorities – particularly with regard to the purpose of education – are considered as sufficiently profound to imply paradigmatic incompatibility. A first attempt to articulate the new paradigm is made and a new model of curriculum development is drawn from development processes implicit in earlier case studies (Chapters 2, 3 and 4).

Within the new paradigm a changed role for nurse education is identified.

INTRODUCTION

Over the last few years, it has been possible to trace ideological shifts in the community of health care educators. A plethora of publications have argued for the rejection of old behaviourist curriculum models. Typically, it is supposed that self-directed learning, critical thinking, action research, reflection on experience (to mention but a few) will, through producing a better practitioner, improve the quality of patient care. In North America, at least, it has been argued that such ideas applied by health care educators have constituted a 'curriculum revolution' (Watson, 1988; Tanner, 1990).

However, as Clare (1993) has recently suggested, it is easier to create a 'curriculum revolution' in the literature than it is to change the practices of health care institutions and their professional employees. Nevertheless, not surprisingly, many authors cling to the notion that changes in curriculum are significant in the wider context. For educators of professionals, this must mean changes in that practice for which they are preparing their students. Yet it is by no means clear that education alone can achieve such ends and indeed there has sometimes been evidence to suggest the contrary (e.g. Menzies, 1960). As Clare observed, the literature of nurse education frequently neglects the context of professional practice, as if health care education was an academic exercise divorced from the political environment in which it in fact must operate. As Ellsworth (1989) has shown, the aspirations of education can be defeated by a clinical orthodoxy. It can be argued that such curriculum 'revolutions' may be at best insubstantial or at worst irrelevant in the context of professional health care practice.

Professional education then cannot be argued in any real sense to be undergoing revolutionary change, unless there is concurrent and significant change in practice. Furthermore, since we have questioned the possibility of education-led changes in practice, we must enquire as to the circumstances in which revolution can occur at all. The answer to this question constitutes the main theme of this book.

As we have argued in Chapter 1, it is our belief that a revolution in health care education is indeed occurring but that it has been triggered by NHS reorganization. In this argument, the political and ideological climate of health care delivery is not just an important component of, or context for, educational change – it is the origin and driving force of it. In this situation, educators are beginning to act in different ways, consider new values and work from new ideologies – in short, to operate within what can loosely be described as a new paradigm.

PROFESSIONAL AND CORPORATE IMPERATIVES

I have referred above to the belief, commonly held by educators, that they are collectively the determinators of practice. The extent to which this notion is implicit in the literature is remarkable. Educationalists repeatedly describe how their ideas and operations can improve the practice of the profession. The confusion here is perhaps due to a faulty extrapolation from the individual student to the profession as a whole. Since educators do produce skilled individual health care professionals, it is a small step to assume that education determines professional practice. In fact, of course, as professional health care educators are largely selected from the ranks of the health care professions, it is easier to identify a mechanism whereby the profession is the dominant influence on practice. It can be argued therefore that education, through a circular process of initiation and socialization, perpetuates a closed system of values and methods of operation, which is analogous to a Kuhnian paradigm as described in Chapter 1. I will therefore now consider some of these professional values and contrast them with the business imperatives of the new NHS trusts.

Spurgeon (1993) has identified the NHS as an organization that has been effective in resisting attempts to change it. He describes the NHS as a 'provider-dominated organization' in which professional views of the appropriateness of services have remained paramount and in which aspects of its nature and structure have enabled professional groups to powerfully resist changes (even when not consciously antagonistic to them). The creation of the internal market and with it the setting up of 'purchasers' has been regarded by Ham (1991) as providing a potential counterbalancing force to this provider power.

The idea of a provider-dominated NHS in which professional views are paramount raises various issues for education and training and so will be considered further. How, for example, has such a situation developed? Some insights may be derived from a brief review of the concept of 'professional'. For our present purposes, we are particularly interested in the extent to which professionalism carries implied stances with regard to stasis and change.

Most conventional views on the nature of professionals identify them as involved in some sort of theory-based practice. Additional defining attributes of the professional are more variable but a number of themes recur in the literature. Typically a level of autonomy among individual practitioners is secured by collective regulation and standard setting within the professional group. The application of high-level knowledge by professionals has led in modern times to the idea of professionals striving to update and improve their services by constant reappraisal of practice in the light of increasingly sophisticated theoretical underpinnings. In this context, the emphasis of education has also shifted, with greater consideration now being given to continuing learning throughout the working life (e.g. Houle, 1980). Such a dynamic concept of the professional has influenced pre-registration courses in nursing, for example, which, as we have seen, are commonly explicitly designed to produce autonomous learners, who are both able and inclined to constantly reflect on and review their practice in the light of experience and research.

Professional autonomy, in so far as it exists, would clearly be a creative force for change if based on such dynamic principles as reflective practice and lifelong learning. Indeed it is hardly debatable that, in the Health Care areas, improvements in clinical practice have resulted from research and reflection on practice by continuously learning professionals. Such improvements, however, derive from within the profession and the concept of professional autonomy may have very different consequences for change whose origins lie outside the professional group.

In institutional terms, the dynamic concept of an internally driven profession has its counterpart in the form of self-regulation and standard-setting. The emphasis here is on professionals as responsible or answerable to their professional peers (through the professional body) rather than any extrinsic accountability. In this context, statutory bodies such as ENB or UKCC can play a similar peer group role. Professionals have therefore long been perceived as being self-organized closed groups (e.g. Flexner, 1915). On the negative side, this collective internal accountability has been interpreted as self-serving and linked with the promotion of social status, mystique and the creation of power bases (Rose, 1974). Illich (1977; 1978) has taken this view further than most.

It is perhaps highly significant in the present context that many analysers of the concept of the professional largely or entirely omit to consider the possibility and implications of their being employed by an organization. Their external responsibility is seen as being direct to the recipient of their services or some concept of society or humanity as a whole.

Where professionals act in independent fee-based practice, the link from individual clients to society as a whole is a simple line relatively unsullied by the complications of employment. On this basis professionals have long been inclined to establish themselves on the moral high ground and to identify 'altruism in motivation' (Flexner, 1915) as one of their characteristics. The existence of an employer, however, can severely compromise this pure concept of professionalism. In circumstances of employment, the context in which professionals operate is subject to other influences and controls. Spurgeon's (1993) link between an NHS resistant to change and the paramountcy of professional views relates to a situation in which desired changes derive from outside the professional groups. In this situation professional groups, in contrast to their otherwise dynamic approach, appear to represent a status quo. We will now consider the position of NHS provider organizations.

The development of the internal market for health services places newly independent health care provider organizations into a new external environment. Such organizations can only secure their future involvement by achieving contracts from purchasers. Furthermore the market implies an element of competition with other prospective providers. Financially independent organizations such as NHS trusts operate within a finite resource, whose size is essentially determined by the combined values of the contracts they successfully obtain. Such organizations must necessarily employ accounting techniques to ensure a sensible relationship between income and expenditure. Financial accounting is not new to health service organizations. However, whereas some pre-reform providers could get by with merely recording the past and present consumption of resources, there is a greater requirement for NHS trusts to predict expenditure in order to take necessary steps to remain solvent. Cost accounting techniques are therefore increasingly used to analyse the costs of future activity and produce financial forecasts. Such financially independent organizations operating in a competitive market (albeit internal and managed) must make large scale decisions that secure their position through combinations of advantageous activities. Coming to these decisions is the business of strategic planning.

In simple terms, strategic planning derives from monitoring the organization's external business environment as well as its available resources and competences. For organizations that can articulate broad and long-term commitments, a 'Mission Statement' could be a third influence. Strategic planning involves an analysis of the situation of the organization, and from this various alternatives may emerge. Examples of this process have recently been reported by our colleagues in the University of Greenwich Business School. The managers of one inner London NHS trust, in examining their environment, recognized that as a consequence of government policy, contracts would move from the acute sector into community budgets. Additionally they recognized that an effect of the internal market would be the loss of certain acute contracts to suburban hospitals that could work more cheaply. A major internal feature of the trust was a chronic lack of capital funds that was not alleviated in the move to trust status. In this situation, the trust managers identified two possible alternative strategic responses: to raise revenue by securing new contracts or to cut provision and its consequent expenditure. An analysis of the feasibility of these alternatives led the trust to pursue the second option – a process that will take years and much detailed planning to implement (Baeza, Salt and Tilley, 1993).

In this example, one trust is cutting provision, while another (suburban) trust has gained new business – for them there is the prospect of additional revenue. Whatever the problems or opportunities created by the internal market, the point to recognize is that such organizations are purposive. They are relatively independent and strive to achieve their ends through the deployment of their resources in the best possible way. These desired ends normally include continued involvement in the provision of quality health care.

Most strategic issues arise from the external environment, and the more fluid or volatile that environment, then the more dynamic the organization must be. Strategic planning in the current NHS internal market implies a systematic approach to change designed to ensure the viability of the organization. The sorts of processes described above convey something of the dynamic nature of 'corporate' organizations. In the current NHS internal market, these organizations are likely to be making rapid strategic responses based on issues of financial viability through a competitive contracting system. Underlying these systems and processes are values far removed from those typically held by health care professionals.

We have seen that, whereas professionals may be highly innovative in clinical practice, many aspects of professionalism suggest complex and tenacious value systems. These have in the past been established on a (false) assumption of care hardly limited by financial constraints. Add to this the prospect of strategic responses involving (intentionally or otherwise) the erosion of professional power bases or radical skills reprofiling and the potential for conflict within provider organizations can be seen to be great. It is not surprising therefore to find one senior manager complaining of senior professionals 'holding up' the process of organizational change (Nettel, 1993).

THE PURPOSE OF EDUCATION AND TRAINING

I have above contrasted professional group characteristics with strategic organizational imperatives. In doing this, I have identified certain value and priority differences which I believe contribute to the tensions in NHS trusts, and which Spurgeon and others feel impede the development of these organizations. This conflict between the professional and the strategic can be seen further reflected in the process of, and attitudes to, education.

Houle (1980) identified the training of professionals to characteristically include 'deep immersion in a specialized content and the acquisition of difficult skills and a complex value system'. This process he regards as being reinforced by experience (e.g. in a hospital) 'which separates the individual from the general public and permeates her thoughts with a distinctive point of view'. As we have mentioned above, the training of the modern professional nurse potentially at least produces dynamic innovation in terms of clinical practice but additionally s/he receives a 'complex value system and distinctive point of view'. It is in the acquisition of this value system that conflict with employers can arise.

In learning to become a professional nurse, a pre-registration student acquires a range of skills and knowledge appropriate to that role. Additionally the student nurses develop a view of themselves as nurses. In terms of Mead's (1934) social psychological analysis, the students concept of 'self' (i.e. the inner and private view that an individual has of her/himself) changes as a consequence of learning to become a nurse, i.e. the student acquires self-identification with the role. This occurs through a process of socialization.

Working in the 1960s, Simpson (1967) identified the socialization of an adult into an occupational role as a sequential process occurring in three analytically distinct stages. The first phase involves a shift from the layperson's view of nurse to the profession's view. Simpson's work showed that in the 1960s the school of nursing at which she studied accomplished this transformation by emphasizing the mastery of technical skills and knowledge (rather than the nurturing of patients which has dominated the students' lay concept of nurse). The second stage of socialization involved the student coming to share other hospital personnel's orientation towards the work situation. Whereas initially the student nurses had considered the patients as 'significant others' in the work situation, the commencement of clinical training had the effect of shifting the student orientation into line with other hospital personnel with whom they developed relationships and attachments. Finally the third stage involved the adoption by the student of behaviour and values presented by the occupational group.

Simpson's work revealed that the college and the clinical area contributed in consistent ways to the development of the professional. For instance, the first-stage shift from the lay person's to the professional's view of nursing was developed by the fact that neither college work or clinical work emphasized nurturing (the college emphasized theory while the clinical work emphasized techniques). Whereas Simpson's work may not represent the present-day practices of nurse education, it does illustrate how the education of a professional nurse involves a process of socialization into current values and practices, and how college tutors and placement staff can effectively collaborate in this process. It is inevitable in such circumstances that the training of nurses tends to generate a new cohort broadly showing the values of the established professionals. In the context of in-house training of nurses (in the sense identified in Chapter 6 where DHA colleges trained for DHA hospitals) whose role is basically stable, such processes of socialization present few real issues and are relatively unproblematic.

Consider, however, the position of a rapidly changing role for nurses in which not only skills and knowledge but also certain professional values are in a process of change. By what means, for example, can the idea of the delivery of health care in the context of a finite resource be taught to student nurses, who must learn skills and values that their predecessors and indeed teachers have not needed to employ? The implications of such changes for nurse education are significant.

It is the employer's perception of education and training that I wish now to consider. Management literature on education and training, whether prior to employment (pre-service) or during employment (in-service) tends to explicitly or implicitly link it with consequent benefit (via the employee) to organizational objectives. Such matters, however, are not considered only in relation to what might be called technical competence. Those involved in the recruitment and selection of staff, for example, are commonly advised to consider how new members of staff would fit into the cultural and social structure of the organization (e.g. Mullins, 1993). Such comments are of particular interest in the area of pre-registration nurse education since organizational culture as commonly defined includes, among other things, values, beliefs and attitudes (McClean and Marshall, 1993) that permeate the organization. As health service provider organizations move into an internal market, certain values are likely to shift and with them over time aspects of organizational culture. Mullins also advises investigation into the potential of prospective appointees, including their flexibility and adaptability to possible new methods, procedures or working conditions. Such ideas in management textbooks are by no means novel; furthermore it is reasonable to suppose that service provider managers, when recruiting health care professionals, look for a composite of skills, values and flexibilities consistent with their perception of the development of the organization.

In-service training of staff in organizational terms is generally seen as an integral part of quality management. Its purpose is considered to be to improve knowledge and skills and 'improve attitudes' (Mullins, 1993). Although recognized as being given low priority in many organizations, it is seen at best as linked to the strategic priorities of the organization (Fill and Mullins, 1990). Thus it is considered a key support system for change and an investment in the long-term survival of the organization. Furthermore, there is evidence that these general ideas are informing the responses of managers. A senior health service manager has, for example recently reported introducing training initiatives related to strategy, market, culture and overall organizational changes, through which every member of staff is clear about her/his role (Nettel, 1993).

In short, employers identify instrumental purposes for education and training. Their priorities relate to quality and the strategic development of their organization and it is generally recognized that education and training is important in relation to values and attitudes, as well as knowledge and skills.

In comparing professional groups and employing organizations in terms of their attitudes to education and training, it is interesting to note that both groups (at least in the literature) attach great importance to education and training but with very different emphasis. Whereas organizational managers identify education and training as a major influence on the success of organizations, professional groups see it as a means of entry into the profession or as a means of upgrading and modernizing knowledge and clinical skills. These different emphases are of course not mutually exclusive. However they do represent ideological differences which in conventional curriculum theory implies different approaches to education and training.

CURRICULUM IDEOLOGIES

Ideology has been defined as a set of related ideas and values held by individuals and groups (OU, 1976). Scrimshaw (1983) has emphasized the role of ideologies as a basis for the determination of the actions of those who hold them. Even in the compulsory sectors of education, school curricula are specified in line with the prevailing ideology of groups with power. This is an important point, since literature on curriculum ideologies is sometimes taken to imply that the prevailing ideology is established by teachers, who apply their beliefs in the design of curriculum. Even in health care education, where teachers have considerable direct control over curriculum design, the prevailing educational ideology is established increasingly by groups external to the teaching community, exerting power. Pendleton (1991) has expressed the view that 'reconstructionist' ideology (Chapter 2) is most relevant to nurse education since nurses, due to their position and experience can be at the forefront of those who work for social justice. This view exemplifies the professional as opposed to corporate priorities identified earlier. Although most educators probably have beliefs and values which are or could constitute an ideology, the beliefs of individuals or even groups of individuals do not necessarily represent a prevailing (i.e. dominant) ideology. In fact, just as in school education, the prevailing educational ideology is the one held by groups with sufficient collective power to exert the predominant influence. In the case of nurse education, analyses in earlier chapters of this book reveal a market for education in which, increasingly, purchasing decisions will be under the influence of health care provider organizations. In the context of education the employer's ideology, as we have seen, is generally instrumental in nature. Employers must necessarily concern themselves primarily with the impact of education and training on their ability to deliver patient care and to develop as organizations.

In this context, the ideologies that may be held by nurse educators, although of interest are of real significance only in terms of the extent to which they correspond to the prevailing ideology. Where there is a profound mismatch between the prevailing ideology and the ideology of a nurse educator, problems can develop. These I will discuss later. Similarly curriculum theorists inclined to compose models and recommend approaches to curriculum development without first identifying the ideological environment in which the curricula must operate are also neglecting important realities. For these reasons I will restrict myself to types of response for an educational climate in which instrumental ideologies are politically ascendent.

Scrimshaw (1983) has made distinctions between what he calls traditional and adaptive instrumentalism. Although his analysis relates to schooling and the needs of society in terms of a skilled workforce, it is also of some interest in the present context. Traditional instrumentalism assumes a relatively stable situation and implies an emphasis on defined vocational skills. Conversely, adaptive instrumentalism identifies complex and changing situations in which specific skills will become obsolete. The emphasis therefore shifts to accommodate those skills which are required across a range of situations (defined as 'transferable' skills) or those which contribute to the individual's ability to actively adjust and develop her/his skills to make them applicable in the new situation (defined by Annett, 1989 as 'transfer skills').

Adaptive instrumentalism is taken by Scrimshaw to imply classroom activities such as group work, guided discussion, problem solving etc. However, although adaptive instrumentalism may often be associated with such approaches, there is no logical necessity for this to follow. Wellington's 1989 conception of 'deferred instrumentalism' (Wellington, 1993) is instructive in this context. This idea derives from the observation that many employers preferentially recruit on the basis of purely 'academic' qualifications. In so far as they see these as indicating general transferable and transfer skills, the ideological background may be described as adaptive instrumentalist. However, such academic qualifications may not have been achieved on the basis of group work, guided discussion and problem solving approaches.

In order to make some progress in this area, I would like, for the purposes of debate, to describe a form of instrumentalism derived explicitly from our earlier analysis of the situation in health care education.

As NHS trusts are formed, the education of nurses increasingly prepares or enhances the ability of a professional to operate in a 'corporate' setting. This, as we have discussed, carries implications for education and training. Notably education and training is increasingly seen as explicitly linked to organizational needs including service quality and organizational development. Since trusts are independent financial organizations, which must compete for business, implied values include working within financial constraints. This leads to values relating to cost-effectiveness, efficiency, etc., as well as the ethical values traditionally associated with health care services. Since education and training is seen as linked to organizational development, it should be a force for change not stasis. For example, in the case of strategic planning including skills reprofiling of

professional groups or delivery by practitioners of health care in a finite budgetary setting, education and training would be contributing to these changes. In
organizational terms, it would be incoherent to purchase education and training
that did not assist with these things.

An ideological stance, which is instrumental and identifies these explicit links
between education and the quality, efficiency and development of an independent organization, I will identify as 'corporate instrumentalism'. Corporate
instrumentalism has some similarities to both traditional and adaptive instrumentalism. On the one hand, it implies certain specific features of education and
training, including understanding of resourcing and costs but, although these
may be considered as specific vocational skills, they are largely transferable.
However it is distinct in its implied focus on the needs of individual
organizations.

Whereas 'corporate instrumentalism' is an ideological position informing employers' views on education and training, it is rarely significant in vocational education. This is because most vocational and professional education is not
directly linked into the specific needs of individual corporate organizations;
rather its purpose is to provide a national workforce from which employers
select. In this context, employers merely provide advice (through advisory committees and so forth), they are not involved in contracting of education. Chapter
6, however, has identified health care education as unique in the extent to which
local employers are actually involved in contracting. Therefore the connection
between the specific (and strategic) needs of the employer can be seen as a feasible and legitimate influence on education. In these circumstances, corporate instrumentalism becomes the dominating ideology and must be the ideological
basis for effective models of curriculum development. (See Silver and Brennan,
1988 for a detailed analysis of the spectrum of links between education and
workforce supply.)

CURRICULUM AS PRODUCT

Earlier parts of this book have analysed and described what is essentially a
market for education. In this market, education provider organizations offer services to purchasers. Chapters 6 and 7 have shown some of these purchasers as
increasingly inclined to devolve purchasing decisions to consortia of NHS trusts.
In any event trusts' influence over education is increasing. In this new environment, education providers tend to lie outside the NHS (as corporate universities)
and therefore we have the organizational financial and legal distinction between
purchaser and provider, which constitutes the main characteristic of the market.
For education providers, such a radically changed environment is demanding
new approaches. In particular, the onus is on the provider to ensure effective relationships with the purchaser. This interface between purchaser and provider
falls within the domain of the business discipline called 'marketing' and it is

from the established theories of marketing that we can find useful practices for the future of health care education.

The purpose of marketing is to enable or facilitate voluntary and mutually advantageous exchange relationships. In our case, 'exchange' refers to the purchasing of educational services, through which colleges achieve revenue, and the output of colleges (skilled practitioners), through which purchasers achieve workforce supply.

The word 'marketing' is wrongly sometimes associated by some with illegitimate exchanges, in which coercion or deceit bring about normally one-off exchanges unsatisfactory to the purchaser. In fact, such techniques have never been a part of marketing proper and today they represent the antithesis of the modern marketing concept, which identifies purchaser satisfaction as of fundamental importance. A second misconception is the widely held belief that marketing equates to advertising or promotional activity. In fact, this represents a milder version of the misconception above, in that both involve a sales orientation in which otherwise insufficient demand is boosted by increasing sales-related activity. There are, however, circumstances in which advertising can indeed create a new market or lead to increased demand. But in health care education this possibility is closed off to an unusual degree since (as Stanwick has discussed in Chapter 7) the purchasing of pre-registration education is explicitly (although not always accurately) matched to employer demand based on workforce analysis.

Whereas educational organizations are generally not inclined to adopt coercion or deceit, they are, in our experience, sometimes prone to adopt a sales orientation rather than address the nature of their services as marketing proper would compel them to do (Humphreys, 1993). Although promotional activity is a legitimate part of marketing, its success will depend on the idea, at the very heart of marketing, that colleges should provide services that purchasers want to buy, rather than trying to persuade them to buy what they choose to provide.

Clearly marketing fits well with instrumental ideologies. Consider an organization and its purchasers. Both have reasons for their interaction. The selling organization achieves its goals and the customers will remain only as long as the product or services satisfies their requirements. The system depends on and therefore encourages mutual satisfaction. This is the conception of marketing that I will apply. In so far as it is overtly instrumental, it is clear and unambiguous and if, at worst, it leads organizations sometimes to confuse self-interest and altruism, this probably happens no more often in purchaser-oriented corporate colleges than it does in professional bodies.

The modern idea of marketing emerged in the 1950s. Recognition of the importance of marketing to education institutions has grown during the 1980s as they have, like NHS trusts, gained autonomy and financial independence (see Chapter 6). Despite an increased profile for marketing in post-compulsory education and training (see for example Davies and Scribbens, 1985; Theodossin, 1989) there is still a great inclination to apply it in limited ways which, while they may improve consumer satisfaction, they may not profoundly affect the service. Such valuable but limited responses include attention to student facilities and corporate image.

The real 'product' of an education provider, however, is learning as experienced by students, i.e. the curriculum in operation. For the student this will contribute significantly to her/his competence, employability and/or professional development. For the employer it can contribute, as we have seen, to the quality of service and strategic development. The most important effect of marketing therefore is the effect is has on the curriculum.

Even in commercial corporate organizations, marketing is by no means a universal philosophy. Doyle (1987) for example found that only 50% of firms he studied developed a genuine consumer orientation. For education organizations, a marketing orientation is not easy to achieve. In particular, it can challenge many conventions (and ideologies). There is, for example, a widely held inclination amongst nurse educators to focus on internal priorities when developing and operating their services. Such internal priorities may involve the ascendancy in curriculum development of epistemological commitments over client needs. For example, a lecturer insisting on a lot of biology in a pre-service curriculum could be asserting this on the basis of genuine customer orientation. Alternatively, he might be doing it because he was a biologist or because he took a liberal, humanist, ideological stance in which science was considered 'important'.

This example illustrates the challenges that marketing creates. Unwillingness to respond to client needs can also be revealed by the use of curriculum dogma (e.g. misused concepts of coherence and progression to put unnecessary limits on flexibility) or a reluctance to tackle operational issues that appears to favour the status quo (e.g. 'it can't be timetabled'). Common to all the curriculum case studies (Chapters 3, 4 and 5) is a disinclination to observe such conventions.

The need to improve the match between employer need and vocational curricula is not new. While the non-advanced further education sector has been encouraged for some time to become more responsive to employment needs (see for example, Cribb *et al.*, 1989), higher education is, particularly through the development and operation of credit accumulation and transfer schemes, recognizing a changed role in the education of professionals (see for example, THES, 1992).

In the general area of professional and vocational training, various authors have given consideration to the significance, in marketing terms, of students and employers. Gray (1989), for example, distinguishes between the two by referring to students as 'customers' and employers as 'clients'. Whether or not students are employees, professional education and training must prepare them to fulfil competently a professional role in an employing organization. Regardless of vocational area, professional courses will at best resolve many apparent conflicts that arise between student and employer need.

It is also important for colleges to formulate a concept of quality which accommodates the clients on which they depend. A key element in any client-sensitive concept of quality will be the match between needs and provision. This apparently simple relationship represents the heart of the marketing idea. Although many colleges would claim a good match, it is very often less apparent to the outside observer than they might think. Current practice appears often to relate provision to needs as perceived in the minds of curriculum developers rather than actual needs. However even national boards (albeit inconsistently) are starting to make the link between quality and the 'corporate objectives' of service providers (ENB, 1990).

While NHS trusts increasingly express concern over the relevance and costs of conventional health care education, many nurse educators, in the absence of any real alternative, practise curriculum development in line with anachronistic but still prevalent methods. While health care itself has shifted to a client-centred stance, health care education struggles with essentially conventional systems of values, beliefs and practices. A nurse tutor, for example, resorting to standard texts on curriculum and curriculum development will find little or no guidance on marketing in relation to curriculum design and, despite some theoretical consideration of instrumentalist curriculum models, no mention of clients (in the sense of NHS trusts).

Yet the situation in health care education now demands a synthesis capable of resolving marketing and the more valuable elements of conventional curriculum theory (Humphreys, 1993). In attempting to begin such a synthesis, I will now consider the marketing equivalent of the practice of curriculum development.

In marketing terms the concept of the 'product' refers to more than simply the basic nature of what is being sold. To the purchaser the 'product' represents a combination of perceived benefits that will meet her/his needs. In designing a product, care is taken to ensure that the full range of the product's attributes are collectively sufficient to interest the purchaser. In educational terms these attributes include the availability of the course (time, location, frequency, etc.) and the price. In marketing terms, the range of attributes associated with a product is referred to as the 'marketing mix'. On the basis of knowledge of the market, including competitor positions, the marketing mix is adjusted in such a way as to best match the product's attributes with identified purchaser needs.

From the case studies described in Chapters 3, 4 and 5, it is possible to abstract certain generic features of the 'curriculum as product' which together constitute a more or less desirable collection of attributes for the purchaser.

Coverage

From the purchaser's point of view, the primary purpose of a course of professional education generally relates to the professional abilities acquired through participation. It is presumed that after participation the learner can do something new or do something better. What it is that s/he is supposed to learn or improve constitutes coverage. The justification for that coverage must derive from the actual or anticipated clinical and other demands in the workplace. For example, a new nurse expected to give intravenous injections immediately on appointment should be equipped with the appropriate knowledge and skills during the course. Although aspects of coverage are established for pre-registration courses by statutory bodies, there remains considerable opportunity for local focus. However it is likely that coverage will remain largely within the control of the educator, rather than the student. In post-registration learning, the professional her/himself may be in a position to partly or wholly determine coverage. Some award-bearing programmes recognize this by leaving coverage entirely open for negotiation.

Coverage may be expressed in various technical formats. Increasingly 'standards', competence statements or learning outcomes are replacing conventional content-laden syllabuses. In any event, a marketing orientation would imply that coverage should be expressed in sufficiently non-technical specification to be accessible to the purchaser.

A recent empirical investigation into trust chief executive views on education (Humphreys, Stanwick and Wood, 1993) identified the match between coverage and future (as opposed to existing) needs to be an important aspect of the quality of education, a point which illustrates the strategic priorities of trust managers in times of change.

Process

By this is meant the processes by which learning is facilitated. Experienced educators often link the process of learning to the desired outcome. This is considered particularly important for the development of professionals as relatively autonomous lifelong learners. In fact, distinct ideologies revolve round the relative importance of content and process. At best, however, in the day-to-day functions of the professional teacher it is not considered an ideological debate. For some hard-pressed clinical practitioners, there may be times where a simple transfer of distilled information may be the most effective approach a teacher can adopt.

Systems

For want of a better word, 'system' is used to describe the range of curriculum structures and facilities from which a curriculum developer must select. These range from an orthodox simple linear sequence through spiral and modular curricula to credit systems with the potential for enormous variability in the way two consumers achieve comparable ends (or indeed different negotiated ends).

Patterns of contact

Contact here refers to face-to-face interaction between student and teacher. In orthodox timetabled programmes a key issue may be the extent to which the timing and pattern of contact provides for easy access. This can be important in both pre- and post-registration education, for some students because of increasingly non-traditional career paths (ENB, 1990) and for others because of pattern of work demand (such as night shifts). Additionally the overall design times of a course (in terms of class contact rather than learning time) and the time interval (or intervals) over which it can be done, are important aspects of curriculum as product.

Learning resources

Appropriate provision of learning resources may take a range of forms from study space and library resources through computer hardware and software to distance learning materials and, of course, access to clinical areas.

Location

Although it is conventional to operate on college premises, alternative approaches are increasingly being taken. Chapter 4, for example, illustrates how a degree level programme of professional development can be achieved through a combination of distance learning and shorter courses based in clinical settings.

Assessment

Conventional curriculum ideologies link approaches to assessment with aspects of process. However even some sacred cows of assessment are being re-examined. The move to competences within NVQ developments has led to the complete detachment of summative assessment from the learning process, with the result that 'assessment on demand' is now considered as a reasonable and normal service to offer to consumers. A more robust link is enshrined in the curriculum concept of assessment 'validity' which links assessment to the nature of the acquired learning (i.e. coverage). Thus, it is considered invalid to assess clinical skills only through written examinations, since written examinations can only test certain components of clinical skills.

Price

Although pricing must ensure that income covers costs, since different approaches carry different costs, there is considerable scope for manipulating other features (e.g. patterns of contact) of curriculum design in order to allow the best combination of attributes.

It is essential to appreciate that none of these features of the curriculum can be seen in isolation. For example, location can interact with learning resources and pattern of contact and coverage can imply process. In fact all eight features can interact in line with the constraints and priorities of the curriculum developer. In a marketing context, the manipulation of these various attributes to produce the best possible combination for the client, represents a new and challenging aspect of curriculum development.

This complex concept of 'product' results in product development procedures that typically include location, price, etc. as an integral rather than peripheral part of product development. However, this is in stark contrast to conventional models of curriculum development. As higher education has become a largely corporate endeavour, resource issues are seen increasingly as a necessary element of the curriculum development process. However this idea has not yet penetrated the literature. Even quite recent textbooks on curriculum and curriculum development fail to make this link (e.g. Pendleton and Myles, 1991; Allen and Jolley, 1987) with the result that there is little appropriate guidance now available for curriculum developers.

A NEW MODEL FOR CURRICULUM DEVELOPMENT

The model of curriculum development identified here has, over the last five years, become implicit in the work of the School of Post Compulsory Education and Training (PCET) at the University of Greenwich. The School is exclusively involved in professional level education and training and operates in a range of market situations. Common to all our work is a need to persuade employers to either use our services directly or to employ our trained output from pre-service programmes. From an initial involvement in the training of further education lecturers and nurse-tutors, we branched out into nursing, midwifery, physiotherapy and social work. Many of these developments involved collaborations with other organizations and, through these collaborations (illustrated by case studies in Chapters 3 and 4) we learnt new ideas and refined our own developmental expertise. Whereas we have been at the forefront of various national developments, we would not claim originality for many of the ideas we have applied. However, in so far as we have had successes, it has been on the basis of developmental approaches which have emerged from the work of PCET staff teams over the last few years (combined with basic operational skills and good practice).

In making our curriculum development model explicit I have had to include all the major elements which make it balanced and complete. In different developments, different parts of the model need emphasis and some parts can be neglected. Where development is collaborative, the sequence and processes must accommodate the partner organization. In any event, the model presupposes an inclination to succeed through the satisfaction of client needs; a constant search for innovation and improvement; and a reluctance to be constrained by conventional curriculum dogma. The model applies to the development of both new and existing curricula.

For convenience of explanation, the model can be considered to consist of three stages: planning, development and validation. Figure 9.1 shows the complete model.

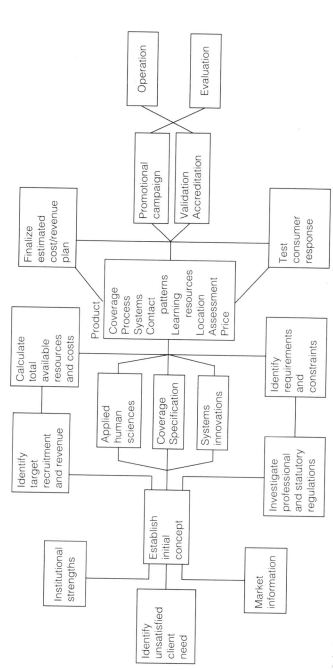

1. Planning 2. Development 3. Validation 4. Operation

Figure 9.1 A model for curriculum development. The largest and central square in the diagram shows the 'curriculum as product' as described in the text. Initial planning is followed by a development stage in which work on resourcing (above) and regulatory issues (below) are seen as distinct from, although in practice integrated with, more orthodox aspects of curriculum development (central strand). A subsequent 'validation' stage involves checking the curriculum design to ensure both positive consumer response and satisfactory cost–price relations. At this point also conventional validation and/or accreditation processes are progressed while a promotional campaign is designed. During the operational stage, evaluation processes monitor fitness for purpose by focusing on client needs as well as the more conventional aspects of educational evaluation. Evaluation feeds into planning and thus a cycle is established.

Planning stage

Planning begins with the identification of an unsatisfied client need. For any organization wishing to diversify, this may have resulted from a systematic search for opportunities. Alternatively, for an existing programme information may derive from employers, students or perhaps increasingly successful competitors.

An initially perceived unsatisfied need generally requires investigating (market information) to ensure firstly, that it is sufficiently widespread to make a response worthwhile, and secondly, that the exact nature of the need is understood. The proposed response in broad terms can be referred to as the 'initial concept'. Although such a concept could be developed *de novo*, it is best, where possible, to apply existing institutional strengths, providing these do not distort the concept beyond the point where it will meet the perceived need.

As an example of this process, we would cite our own collaboration with Macmillan, publishers of *Nursing Times*. The advent of P2000 etc. marked the obsolescence of the enrolled nurse. This position is unsatisfactory for enrolled nurses, many of whom saw conversion to registered nurse as a solution. Market information revealed the level of dissatisfaction to be very great; in some districts it was estimated that, with the current availability of enrolled nurse conversion courses, it would take 10 years to convert the enrolled nurses who wished to do so. Macmillan linked this unsatisfied need to their strength as publishers and set up the Nursing Times Open Learning Scheme (NTOL) which was accredited by all four UK National Boards in 1991. In 1993, NTOL reached agreement with the University of Greenwich School of Post Compulsory Education and Training (PCET) to recognize the NTOL programme as credit towards a higher education qualification. At that time, PCET had developed a strength in the application of credit systems to professional training. PCET aware of a related need for existing registered nurses also to achieve higher education qualifications proposed a linked credit-based development for both markets. It is now possible for both enrolled and registered nurses to work to a University of Greenwich Diploma of Higher Education through Nursing Times Open Learning. Currently over 2000 students are enrolled.

In this case, the concept applied strengths in publishing and in credit schemes to two related and unsatisfied needs. The resulting programmes operate on the basis of distance learning materials published weekly in *Nursing Times*, and support available through approved centres around the UK.

Development stage

The developmental stage consists of three elements, shown in Figure 9.1 as running in parallel but in fact to a large degree integrated. These relate to resourcing and regulatory factors, as well as 'design' features relating to coverage and systems. Each will be considered in turn.

Resourcing

In order to properly establish the nature of resourcing issues that must be considered in the model, it is first necessary to briefly address some background information on the past and future practices of college finance.

Colleges which formed part of district health authorities (Chapter 7) are subject to that organization's financial accounting systems. These systems were designed to keep accurate records of their financial affairs, including expenditure and income. Typically, expenditure on the college would constitute a relatively small part of a large overall DHA annual spend. Furthermore, instead of college expenditure being drawn from special college budgets, it has been the practice with many colleges for expenditure to be drawn from the general budgets of the parent organization. So, for example, salaries of college staff would be drawn from staffing budgets that covered other district employees, while building maintenance, cleaning services, etc. would likewise be covered by district budgets.

In these circumstances a college is not seen as a financially separate part of the DHA and, because of this, there is no comprehensive overall annual figure of total college expenditure. Indeed, even when such a figure is desired, it can be very difficult to get at since most financial information on the college is 'lost' among the millions of pieces of data in the overall DHA financial accounting system.

A college in this position is not of course free from various financial constraints. In particular limits can be put on more easily distinguished college expenditure such as on staffing. Typically a college would have a staff 'establishment' based on some estimate of how many staff would be needed to sustain the education and training function. Student–staff ratio (SSR) could provide the basis for calculating establishments but in fact SSR used in this way is problematic, not least because of numerous variations in the way it can be calculated. Often SSR had provided a rough basis, in addition to which negotiations between a college and its parent organization over particular cases for extra staffing might be argued and sometimes accommodated.

We could refer to this method of resourcing as 'education-led'. Behind it are fairly orthodox educational assumptions about class sizes and methods of teaching and learning. In some colleges it has been the practice to design a curriculum and then calculate the resource needed to run it. If the available resource falls short, then a case is made for more. It has also been common practice in colleges of nursing to argue for extra resourcing for the development of new programmes. This also is a logical request in a system that derives an establishment primarily from estimating what is needed to operate (rather than develop) courses.

In summary, the past (and for some, present) situation is ignorance about the total expenditure of a college and 'education-led' college resourcing systems. We must now compare this with the financial and budgetary system necessary for colleges which are, or form part of independent financial organizations (such as universities).

A limitation of financial accounting is that it is concerned with the past and the present. Expenditure is only known about after it has occurred (or money has been committed). This alone is insufficient for many financially independent organizations which need to anticipate future financial positions. The cost of a service such as a course includes all the money spent on providing it. It is made up of 'direct costs' such as labour and materials together with its apportioned share of overheads such as building maintenance and rent. These latter 'indirect costs' also include a portion of staffing costs for the personnel, finance and other departments not directly involved in the service delivered. In educational organizations it is not uncommon for the indirect costs of a service to be more than the direct costs.

In a market situation the full cost of a service must normally be known in order to establish a price. As we have seen the information about the costs of whole colleges is often hard to achieve and the costs of individual courses are even more remote. In the reorganized NHS, hospital trusts are having very similar problems and it is partly because of this that service contracting is currently negotiated coarsely for large numbers of 'completed consultant incidents'. However contract prices are achieved, they must nevertheless cover costs. If they do not, then the financial viability of the organization may be at risk and drastic measures may need to be taken.

In this context, courses must be designed to operate within a specified resource and curriculum development must include resourcing as an integral part of course design. Since the income to cover costs comes ultimately from the purchaser, the process of curriculum development might be described as 'market-led'.

An organization with adequate cost accounting systems may, through its managers, simply constrain curriculum development groups to design services that can operate within anticipated income, i.e. the relationship between anticipated income and expenditure is clear, explicit and expressed in terms of money. Frequently, however, educational organizations do not yet have sufficiently sophisticated costing systems with the consequence that they identify resources available to courses in currencies other than money. Commonly for example they may determine the staffing resource through an SSR calculation. In this market-led situation, however, SSR is used as the basis of a formula to determine available resource.

The distinction between the uses of SSR in 'education-led' and 'market-led' contexts is subtle but profound. ENB, for example, specify an SSR as a means of ensuring what they consider to be a satisfactory staff level. There is a notional relationship between SSR and class sizes, etc. which is assumed to relate in some way to quality – i.e. SSR is being used to ensure quality. There is no implied knowledge of actual income–expenditure relationships.

On the other hand, in a market-led situation, SSR is used as a means of manipulating the income–expenditure relationship in such a way as to ensure that income covers costs. In these circumstances, a course team is given an SSR from which, combined with target recruitment, it can calculate the total hourage available for the course. For example, if a college knew that, in order to make ends meet, it needed courses in a particular department to run on an SSR of 20:1 then, for each 20 full-time students, one member of staff would be available. If, say, one member of staff could teach 15 hours per week, then 20 students would generate 15 class contact hours and the design team would have to work within this resource (this example is simplified).

To summarize, in an education-led resourcing system, SSR is established on the basis of some idea of quality, and expenditure is a consequence of this. Conversely, in a market-led resourcing system, SSR is established on the basis of anticipated income and quality is derived from the skills of the curriculum developer who must design the course to operate within the anticipated available resource.

Increasingly higher education organizations are moving away from SSR as part of a 'market-led' resource deployment formula, and instead introducing so-called 'cost centres' in which income and expenditure are even more explicitly and directly linked. Here the full costs (direct and indirect) of a course must normally be met by income. In a contracting system, the price is set to at least cover costs. In designing curricula, therefore, a team must consider the collective attractiveness to purchasers of various patterns of attributes: inclusive of price and programme design. There is unlikely to be a long-term benefit in sacrificing basic sufficient quality for reduced prices. However those curriculum development teams who can imaginatively design cost-effective programmes will be highly valuable to their organizations. Such programmes may be highly innovative in design, a possibility we will discuss further below.

Regulations

Because there is nothing new about the need for programmes to comply with various regulations, this section will be kept brief. Such regulations are established by internal and external groups with power, who for various reasons must constrain curriculum development teams or sometimes encourage them to develop in particular directions. Internal regulations in universities are often specified in order to keep a broad consistency in the various programmes offered across the whole organization. Typically they are established by 'academic standards' committees and ensured via the university procedures for course validation. In the new universities, academic standards committees serve a purpose analogous to the former (external) role of the Council for National Academic Awards. They are positioned outside the managerial structure of the university and remain independent of cost centres.

External regulatory organizations include statutory bodies such as the national boards and NCVQ, professional bodies, such as the Chartered Society of Physiotherapists, and curriculum agencies such as BTEC, City and Guilds, etc. Although, in many ways constraining and to some extent inevitably lagging behind the forefront of curriculum design, some are inclined to encourage innovation and, in doing this, can facilitate development in those education providers who need a push. Examples of such facilitation is provided in Chapter 3 and 4 of this book.

In any event, regulations established by such organizations constitute an important part of the environment in which education providers must operate.

Design

As we have seen, regulations, although constraining, generally leave considerable discretion to the curriculum developer. Resource issues, on the other hand, can (depending on the particular college) interact dynamically with other aspects of the product. For instance a lower cost curriculum may require less 'teaching' through class contact with greater emphasis on alternative learning situations. This is by no means a straightforward or easily predictable relationship. The development of learning resources for distance learning, for example, carries considerable development and production costs. Whether or not distance learning approaches carry more or less cost is dependent on parameters including target and actual recruitment, lifespan of the curriculum and specific patterns and extent of tutorial time, classroom use, access to library, etc. Nevertheless, in the increasing number of colleges with adequate cost accounting systems, it is feasible for costs and therefore prices to be one of the variables that developers can manipulate during the curriculum design process. Without this flexible facility cost will be a more static factor but, since it must be limited within anticipated income (directly or through SSR minima), it remains an integral part of curriculum development.

Whatever the cost and regulation circumstances, curriculum developers must make design decisions. In this model the curriculum developer can use her/his professional judgement to assemble the best design elements for the particular situation. From our earlier discussion, we know that design must include: coverage, processes and systems. However, in reality, the three often tend to be highly interdependent. Competences or learning goals, for example, signify both content and learning process. Similarly, APEL and CATS systems can be incompatible with close and tightly sequenced curricula. Nevertheless, there is considerable scope for designing the curriculum to best meet the client needs. Chapter 5 described a curriculum development process that was designed explicitly to accommodate the needs of both the employing organizations and in-service students. Among the various attributes assembled were a combination of competences and learning goals, as this was considered the strongest response to the situation identified in the Planning Stage.

The model (Figure 9.1) identifies three distinct functional elements in the design process: coverage specification; applied human sciences and systems innovations. These will be considered in turn.

In this model, coverage is derived from client need. Whereas this may seem an obvious statement, we have seen that there is a tendency instead amongst curriculum developers to focus on internal priorities derived from non-instrumental ideological stances. Curriculum developers should be careful not to overvalue their own personal views as to what should be included. This can lead to blatantly self-serving priorities (such as the biologist mentioned earlier who emphasizes the importance of biology and argues for more, rather than less, regardless of whether it is appropriate). Even more genuine ideologically derived arguments can take the focus off client need. These may include purely epistemological justifications for 'coherence' or conventional humanist-derived arguments for studies with only peripheral relevance. Such approaches may be appropriate for school education but do little to enhance professional education purchased by employers. Furthermore, in the education of health care professions, the inclusion of secure knowledge bases, ethics, transferable skills, etc. may often legitimately derive from a client-led approach. Where these things are important, this curriculum model will deliver them.

Coverage is sometimes taken to imply fixed sequence. This sort of approach can derive from the behaviourist tradition but also from the otherwise incompatible area of cognitive psychology. In the latter case an analysis of the conceptual structure of a subject may help to identify prerequisite relationships which suggest necessary learning sequences (e.g. Humphreys, 1987) for biology. The idea of necessary sequence, however, can be taken beyond that which conceptual analysis can justify. Where this happens, the unnecessary reduction in curriculum flexibility can run counter to client interests.

Knowles's work on the adult learner and Schon's on the autonomous professional (both discussed in the earlier chapters) have led to more flexible approaches to curriculum design in which the needs of individual learners can be accommodated. In the School of PCET, we have been introducing 'real time' flexibility into curricula, such that professionals in both initial and post-experience training can select units of learning when the work demand requires particular knowledge and skills. In this way, the demand on professionals is matched in terms of both the coverage and timing of particular learning programmes (add to this flexibility of location and the true significance of this approach begins to emerge).

Where prerequisite relationships between concepts/skills, etc. are genuine, then a skilled professional educator will recognize them. Beyond this, however, flexible approaches to content sequence may be beneficial. The best balance may depend on the stage of the individual in her/his training. Certainly pre-registration programmes are likely to be more structured; even here, however, there is much more opportunity than is sometimes appreciated.

The use of conceptual analysis to determine real prerequisite relationships shows how human sciences (in this case psychology) can be applied by the expert educator to enhance the design of curricula. Mike Kelly, a colleague at the University of Greenwich, has recently described an approach to curriculum development, in which explicit instrumental objectives were accommodated into curriculum design by the application of models of behaviour. Kelly and

Maloney (1992) were involved in the development of a health promotion course for nurses. Underlying the course was a concern that stress-related health effects on nurses were impinging on morale, turnover, absenteeism, general patient care and the delivery of services. In designing a programme to improve this situation Kelly and Maloney applied a model of stress-coping developed by Lazarus (1980). Lazarus identified coping as consisting of threat recognition followed by a decision about appropriate action. The former is information-based and the latter skill-based. In curriculum terms the implication is that information alone is inadequate. If the objective is a reduction in smoking rates, then in addition to information about the dangers of smoking nurses would also need to develop the necessary skills to give up (Kelly, 1990).

The final element in the curriculum design process relates to systems innovations. By this is meant structural configurations (such as spiral curricula, curriculum stages or parts, modularity, etc.) and system facilities such as flexibility, negotiation, APEL and APL.

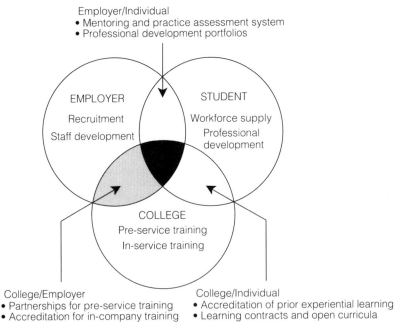

Employer/Individual
• Mentoring and practice assessment system
• Professional development portfolios

EMPLOYER

Recruitment

Staff development

STUDENT

Workforce supply

Professional development

COLLEGE
Pre-service training
In-service training

College/Employer
• Partnerships for pre-service training
• Accreditation for in-company training

College/Individual
• Accreditation of prior experiential learning
• Learning contracts and open curricula

Figure 9.2 Functional links between employer, college and student, with two examples of curriculum systems innovations at each interface. Through pre-service training the college produces a workforce supply for the employer. Recruitment from this pool is followed by ongoing staff development often through in-service training by the college. For the individual this contributes to her/his development as a professional. These functional links can be facilitated by curriculum systems innovations (see text).

Figure 9.2 identifies functional links between the three key players in the education market and six systems innovations which relate to the interfaces between employer, college and student. The three case studies (Chapters 3, 4 and 5) included a range of examples of the application of such facilities.

The fact that in health care education, education providers normally work closely with both employer and student gives them the opportunity to work towards an ideal in which through the operation of programmes, both individual and organizational needs are met. Chapter 5, in particular, described a development which has had some success in resolving the apparent contradictions that sometimes appear to exist between the educational needs of employer and student. In an ideal instrumental, market-led situation, education and training will recognize and work towards meeting the needs of both.

Validation and operation

These last two stages in the curriculum development model involve checking the relationship between client need and curriculum design. Although validation (as a stage in this model) includes normal course validation and/or accreditation procedures it also should involve a check by the development team against the initial concept (articulated in the planning stage) and the anticipated cost–revenue relationship. At best these checks involve potential consumers and purchasers.

Once these things are confirmed a promotional campaign can be developed to ensure that the benefits of the product are communicated to prospective students and/or purchasers. Chapter 5 has illustrated this process.

During the operational stage, evaluation processes should monitor fitness for purpose in addition to conventional aspects of academic and professional standards.

In the health promotion course for nurses considered above Kelly and Maloney (1992) based the approach taken in course evaluation on a model of behavioural change. In this case, a theory of self-development identified success in, for instance, giving up smoking to involve both a 'self-driven' behaviour change combined with a change in social identity (from smoker to non-smoker). Evaluation therefore involved assessment of both the extent to which people came to desire to break the habit and the extent to which they were in fact able to do this. It is interesting here that the instrumental nature of the course was reflected in both development and evaluation. The latter being directly linked to the objectives of the programme rather than just measuring its 'entertainment value and technical operation'.

THE ROLE OF THE PROFESSIONAL EDUCATOR

A major implication of these approaches to education and training is the high levels and range of skills required from professional educators. In addition to systematic and objective ways of identifying necessary coverage, the curriculum developer must ideally have a good working knowledge of costing, applied human sciences, curriculum systems and an inclination to innovate. In addition, the professional educator must contribute effectively to the operation of the resulting programmes and contribute in other ways to the operation and development of the college. This sort of challenge cannot merely be an appendage to the skills of the professional nurse or other health care provider. To be most effective the education professional must perceive her/himself as such.

Many would argue (myself included) that the effective health care educator maintains a direct involvement with patients. However this should no longer be an end in itself but rather a means to an end – that end being to effectively deliver health care education. It is a perennial problem with teachers (at least in post-compulsory education) that they tend to retain a primary affiliation with their first career (engineer, scientist, nurse, etc.) rather than their second (education). This stance may be less problematic in a period of professional stability but is of limited use at times when education could be contributing to significant institutional, professional and organizational change. Bearing in mind the discussions earlier in this chapter, it is not surprising to find professional groups (e.g. RCN, 1993) arguing as if the profession of (for instance) nurse and the profession of educator constituted subsets of one profession. However, as I have argued, it is questionable whether the professional interests of the one are compatible with the change agent role of the other.

Furthermore, the fact that a nurse tutor is not primarily a nurse is not only a matter of professional stance. Increasingly, as nurse education is removed from health authorities, so nurse tutors become legally separated from the organization whose clients are patients. It has been shown in Chapter 7 that the nurse tutor who considers patients to be her/his clients is both rejecting the position of professional educator and exhibiting a misinterpretation of reality. While it is true that the education of health professionals is a critical factor in the delivery of health care to patients, the relationship is indirect and there are in reality only two clients – the students and the employing organizations. This position essentially means that the service provider is increasingly the primary client of the education provider, at least with regard to WP10-funded contracts. A simplistic response to this circumstance would be to suggest that an education provider must do whatever the purchasing client says. However, this presupposes that service providers are in a position to specify the nature of the education services which would meet their needs. It is more likely however that at best they will simply know what they are trying to achieve!

Consider, for example, an advertising agency working for a large corporate organization (the client) in a service industry. Assuming the client organization is well established and internally coherent, it will know exactly what it wants to achieve through advertising (e.g. 5% increase in sales). However, although it may have some required features, it will not be in a position to specify the detailed nature of an advertising campaign, nor would it be in a position to implement it.

Any company that was inclined and able to design, specify and implement the campaign would be unlikely to employ an advertising agency. If over time the agency did indeed contribute effectively to the client's goals, then it would be retained. If it did not, it would be vulnerable and if for some reason it showed little response to the client's priorities, it would certainly lose the contract. In the same way, there is in the new environment an implied onus on education providers to recognize the nature of their relationship with service providers, to understand their goals and difficulties and to come up with education services designed, recommended and operated on the basis of that understanding.

A major and general challenge for the designers of vocational curricula is therefore to identify the needs of the employers. Wellington (1993), having reviewed a number of surveys into employer's perceptions, suggested that 'the needs of employers are complex and not always immediately tangible'. He found their statement of needs to 'contain a conceptual mixture of attributes, qualities, dispositions, attitudes, competences and general skills' and observed that their stated needs did not always coincide with their actual practices. Because of this, superficial attempts at employer liaison through advisory committees or employer involvement in curriculum teams are of little real use except perhaps at strategic level or as public relations (see Chapter 8 for a more profound attempt to keep in touch with clients).

Although the surveys considered by Wellington related to 'industry' in general (i.e. a range of industries) the point is nevertheless valid that organizations rarely have the time or skills to articulate their needs in such a way as to provide an adequate basis for curriculum development. Certain aspects of the situation in health care education would, however, seem to alleviate the problem. Firstly, a consistency of need could derive from the broadly similar occupations found across a range of employers (e.g. nurse, midwife, physiotherapist) and secondly, many of these occupations are professions regulated in various ways by professional and statutory bodies. Educationalists however should be very cautious of deriving reassurance from the professional regulation of occupations. In the first place, there are often an enormous range of possibilities for local focus, which fall within the broad requirements of a professional or statutory body, and secondly, the existence of professional regulation can, for educators trying to identify and respond to corporate needs, create more tensions and difficulties than they solve. As we have seen, resolution of such tensions is a part of curriculum development.

This view of health care education may not please many. Set in an instrumental context, the work is judged on nothing more than its utility. Furthermore the educator is not accountable to patients but to students and client organizations. In Anglo Saxon culture, notions of applied knowledge and utility carry negative connotations (Glover and Kelly, 1987) compared to purely 'academic' pursuits. While health care professionals carry their own special status derived from direct contact with patients, the educator *qua* educator may work only indirectly for patient benefit and, as the role has been articulated here, it might be judged to have been diminished. However, it has been shown that the instrumentally based education and training of corporate professionals is highly demanding. It is based on a multidisciplinary range of skills and knowledge; it requires sophisticated educational practice. There is no place for ideological indulgence, school-derived orthodoxies, sacred cows or anachronistic dogmas. To that extent, at least, the new fire of corporate instrumentalism may be no worse than the old frying pan of institutionalized professional interest. Time will tell.

REFERENCES

Allen, P. and Jolley, M. (eds) (1987) *The Curriculum in Nursing Education*, Chapman & Hall, London.

Annett, J. (1989) *Training in Transferable Skills*, Training Agency, Sheffield.

Baeza, J., Salt, D. and Tilley, I. (1993) Four providers strategic responses and the internal market, in *Managing the Internal Market*, (ed. I. Tilley), Paul Chapman, London.

Clare, J. (1993) Change the curriculum – or transform the conditions of practice. *Nurse Education Today*, **13**, 282–286.

Cribb, M. *et al.* (1989) *Planning a Curricular Response*, Further Education Unit, London.

Davies, P. and Scribbins, K. (1985) *Marketing Further and Higher Education*, Longman for FEU and FESC, Harlow.

Doyle, P. (1987) Marketing and the British Chief Executive. *Journal of Marketing Management*, **3**(2).

Ellsworth, E. (1989) Why doesn't this feel empowering? Working through the repressive myths of critical pedagogy. *Harvard Educational Review*, **59**(3), 297–323.

ENB (English National Board) (1990) *The Collapse of the Conventional Career*, English National Board for Nursing, Midwifery and Health Visiting, London.

ENB (English National Board) (1993) *Guidelines for Educational Audit: Quality Education for Quality Care*, English National Board for Nursing Midwifery and Health Visiting, London.

Fill, C. and Mullins, L.J. (1990) The effective management of training. *Industrial and Commercial Training*, **22**(1), 13–16.

Flexner, A. (1915) Is social work a profession? *School and Society*, **1**, 901–911.

Glover, I.A. and Kelly, M.P. (1987) *Engineers in Britain - A Sociological Study of the Engineering Dimension*, Allen & Unwin, London.

Gray, L. (1989) Marketing education services, in *Educational Institutions and Their Environments*, (ed. R. Glatter), Open University Press, Milton Keynes.

Ham, C. (1991) If it isn't hurting, it isn't working. *Marxism Today*, **July**, 14–17.

Houle, C.O. (1980) *Continuing Learning in the Professions*, Jossey-Bass, London.

Humphreys, J. (1987) The evaluation of fieldwork: concept elucidation by transects. *Journal of Biological Education*, **21**(1), 28–34.

Humphreys, J. (1993) The marketing gap in health care education. *Nurse Education Today*, **13**, 202–209.

Humphreys, J., Stanwick, S., and Wood, K. (1993) *The QUACE Pack: Quality Assurance for Contracting of Education*, South East Thames Regional Health AuthorityJ (Directorate of Nursing and Quality), Kent.

Illich, I. (1977) *Disabling Professions*, Marion Boyars, London.

Illich, I. (1978) *The Right to Useful Unemployment and its Professional Enemies*, Marion Boyars, London.

Kelly, M.P. (1990) A suitable case for technik: behavioural science in the postgraduate medical curriculum. *Medical Education*, **24**, 271–279.

Kelly, M.P. and Maloney, W.A. (1992) A behavioural modelling approach to curriculum development and evaluation of health promotion for nurses. *Journal of Advanced Nursing*, **17**, 544–547.

Lazarus, R. (1980) The stress coping paradigm, in *Competence and Coping During Adulthood*, (eds L. Bond and J. Rosen), University Press of New England, New Hampshire.

McClean, A. and Marshall, J. (1993) *Intervening in Cultures*, University of Bath, Bath.

Mead, G.H. (1934) *Mind, Self and Society*, Chicago University Press, Chicago.

Menzies, I. (1960) *A Case Study in the Functioning of Social Systems as a Defence against Anxiety*, Tavistock Institute of Human Relations, London.

Mullins, L.J. (1993) *Management and Organizational Behaviour*, 3rd edn, Pitman, London.

Nettel, J. (1993) The purchaser/provider split as seen by a major provider: the case of King's Healthcare, in *Managing the Internal Market*, (ed. I. Tilley), Paul Chapman, London.

Open University (1976) *Curriculum Design and Development*, E203, Open University Press, Milton Keynes.

Pendleton, S. (1991) Curriculum planning in nursing education: towards the year 2000, in *Curriculum Planning in Nursing Education*, (ed. S. Pendleton and A. Myles), Edward Arnold, London.

Pendleton, S. and Myles A. (eds) (1991) *Curriculum Planning in Nursing Education*, Edward Arnold, London.

RCN (Royal College of Nursing) (1993) *Teaching in a Different World*, A RCN Discussion Document, Royal College of Nursing, London.

Rose, G. (1974) Issues in professionalism: British social work triumphant, in *A Design for Social Work Practice*, (ed. Perlmutter), Colombia University Press, New York.

Scrimshaw, P. (1983) *Educational Ideologies*. Unit 2 of Educational Studies, E204, Open University Press, Milton Keynes.

Silver, H. and Brennan, J. (1988) *A Liberal Vocationalism*, Methuen, London.

Simpson, I.H. (1967) Patterns of socialization into professions: the case of student nurses. *Sociological Inquiry*, **37**, 47–54.

Spurgeon, P. (1993) Regulation or free market for the NHS? A case for co-existence, in *Managing the Internal Market*, (ed. I. Tilley), Paul Chapman, London.

Tanner, C. (1990) Reflections on the curriculum revolution. *Journal of Nursing Education*, **29**(7), 295–299.

Theodossin, E. (1989) *Marketing the College*, Further Education Staff College, Bristol.

THES (1992) Corporate classroom. *Times Higher Education Supplement*, **3 July**.

Watson, J. (1988) Curriculum in transition, in *Curriculum Revolution: Mandate for Change*, (ed. National League for Nursing), National League for Nursing, New York.

Wellington, J. (ed.) (1993) *The Work Related Curriculum*, Kogan Page, London.

Index

Page numbers in **bold** type refer to **figures** and page numbers in *italic* type refer to *tables*.

Health Psychology

2nd edition

Processes and applications

Edited by **A. K. Broome**, Clinical Psychologist, Weymouth, Dorset, UK, and
S. P. Llewelyn, Department of Psychiatry, University of Edinburgh, UK

The second edition of this successful standard text preserves the strengths of the first edition in its comprehensive coverage of a wide area of application. Some chapters and authors have altered, but the book's overall framework remains the same.

New chapters address the context of health care provision, stress and cardiac disorders. The existing chapters have been extensively updated to include new research material and areas of application. The book presents theory first and application second, stressing the need for a clear understanding of principles before putting psychology into practice.

Features:

● discusses both the theory and application of health psychology

● discusses the major issues in the field

● has a comprehensive discussion of a series of applications of health psychology

Contents: Introduction - *A. Broome and S. Llewelyn*. Health beliefs and attributions
- *T. Marteau*; Stress and health - *T. Cox*; Placebos: their effectiveness and modes of action
- *P. Richardson*; Applying health psychology in health and community care settings - *B. Kat*;
Improving patient's understanding, recall, satisfaction and compliance - *P. Ley and S. Llewelyn*; Institutional versus client-centred care in general hospitals - *K. A. Nichols*; Caring: the costs to nurses and relatives - *S. Llewelyn and S. Payne*; Patients' contributions to the consultation - *E. Robinson*; Cardiac disorders - *C. Bundy*; Dermatology - *P. Janes*; Diabetes mellitus - *R. Shillitoe*; Psychological aspects of physical disability - *S. Wilkinson*; Gastroenterology - *P. Bennet*; General practice: the contribution of clinical psychology
- *I. McPherson*; Geriatric medicine - *N. Bradbury*; Gynaecology - *M. Hunter*; Psychological aspects of neurological illness - *L. Earll*; Emotional factors in hearing loss - *S. Jakes*;
Obstetrics - *L. Sherr*; Paediatrics and childhood cancer - *N. Whitehead*; Chronic pain
- *A. Erskine and A. C. de C. Williams*; Renal care - *C. G. Long*; Surgery - *J. Kincey*; Terminal care - *C. Wilson*; Index.

September 1994: 246x189: c.448pp, 12 line illus; paperback: 0 412 55120 9: £24.99

CHAPMAN & HALL

Principles and Practice of Nurse Education

3rd edition

F. M. Quinn, Healthcare Education Department, University of Greenwich, UK

This successful book has been revised to include the many changes in nurse education. It is the only book that covers the complete spectrum of education as applied to nursing and healthcare professions.

From a review of the second edition:
'For student teachers in nursing, I highly recommend this book. It will also be very beneficial to qualified teachers for updating or to others seeking an understanding of the complex issues involved in the theory and practice of nurse education.' *Nursing Standard*

Features:

- revised, with new chapters to meet today's educational needs

- reflects the move to higher education

- educational approach covers the whole field of adult education

- new chapters include: planning for teaching, quality assurance, educational delivery systems, course management

- the examples given are from nursing, but they apply to any aspect of adult education, particularly to health science disciplines

Contents: Educational psychology: cognitive approaches. Educational psychology: behaviourist and other approaches. Educational psychology: individual differences, social influences and motor skills. Study skills and strategies. Lecturing. Small-group teaching. Practice-based learning. Information technology and media resources. Educational delivery systems. The curriculum: principles and organisation. Assessment. Educational quality assurance. Course management. Tutoring and counselling. Teaching biological concepts. Teaching communication skills. Research and enquiry in nurse education. Index.

September 1994: 246x189: c.496pp, 44 line illus; paperback: 0 412 43550 0: c. £17.50

CHAPMAN & HALL

Health Education

2nd edition

K. Tones and **S. Tilford,** Leeds Metropolitan University, UK

Since the first edition of this book was published, in 1990, health promotion has been enjoying an increasingly high profile both nationally and internationally. For this new edition, many chapters have been extensively revised or rewritten to take account of recent developments. New issues about health education are discussed and, as a result, the book provides a more comprehensive and critical review of health promotion and its relationship with health education.

In addition to presenting detailed analysis of different models of health education and discussing implications for evaluation, a greater emphasis has been placed on the values and ideological issues permeating attempts to assess the effectiveness and efficiency of health education. The book argues the case for critically appraising the implicit and explicit values and associated ethical issues which are central to the process of evaluation. It also reiterates the importance of grounding evaluative research and health education programmes on a firm, explicit and coherent foundation of theory.

From a review of the first edition:
'Books on health education can easily be wishy washy, uninspirational and unscientific, but this is not one of them. . . This book will be useful for all those concerned with health and social policy, particularly in health promotion, prevention, and public health.'

British Medical Journal

Features:

- addresses current issues within health education including the impact of environmentalism to keep the reader well informed

- paperback, reduced price and therefore suitable for the student market

- the standard work, revised and updated for current courses

- illustrated by models and figures for ease of reference

Contents: Introduction. **Part One:** The meaning of success. Indicators of success and the meaning of performance. Research design in evaluation: Choices and issues.
Part Two: School health education. Health care contexts. Mass media in health education. Health promotion in the workplace. Community organization and strategic integration: Promoting community health. Index.

April 1994: 234x156: 336pp, 29 line illus; paperback: 0 412 55110 1: £19.99

CHAPMAN & HALL